THE STRUGGLE OF BLIND PEOPLE
FOR SELF-DETERMINATION

ABOUT THE AUTHOR

Ed Vaughan received his B.A. degree from West Virginia University and a M.Div. from Union Theological Seminary, New York. He received his M.A. and Ph.D. degrees in Sociology from the University of Minnesota.

For the past twenty-three years he has been a member of the faculty at the University of Missouri-Columbia. He has served as chair of the Department of Sociology and as Director of the Center for Research on Aging. He currently holds the rank of Professor in the Department of Sociology at the University of Missouri-Columbia.

In 1991, Professor Vaughan was a visiting Professor at Xi'An Foreign Languages University, People's Republic of China. He returned to China in the summer of 1992 to continue his research on programs for disabled people in China.

THE STRUGGLE OF BLIND PEOPLE FOR SELF-DETERMINATION

The Dependency-Rehabilitation Conflict: Empowerment in the Blindness Community

By

C. EDWIN VAUGHAN, PH.D.

Professor, Department of Sociology
University of Missouri
Columbia, Missouri

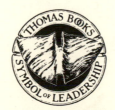

CHARLES C THOMAS • PUBLISHER
Springfield • Illinois • U.S.A.

Published and Distributed Throughout the World by

CHARLES C THOMAS • PUBLISHER
2600 South First Street
Springfield, Illinois 62794-9265

© *1993 by* CHARLES C THOMAS • PUBLISHER

ISBN 0-398-05854-7

Library of Congress Catalog Card Number: 93-20088

With THOMAS BOOKS *careful attention is given to all details of manufacturing
and design. It is the Publisher's desire to present books that are satisfactory as to their
physical qualities and artistic possibilities and appropriate for their particular use.*
THOMAS BOOKS *will be true to those laws of quality that assure a good name
and good will.*

Printed in the United States of America
SC-R-3

Library of Congress Cataloging-in-Publication Data

Vaughan, C. Edwin.
    The struggle of blind people for self-determination : the
dependency-rehabilitation conflict : empowerment in the blindness
community / C. Edwin Vaughan.
    p.   cm.
    Includes bibliographical references and index.
    ISBN 0-398-05854-7
    1. Blind—Rehabilitation—United States. 2. Blind—
Rehabilitation—Economic aspects—United States. 3. Blindness—
Psychological aspects. I. Title.
HV1795.V38   1993
362.4′18′0973—dc20   93-20088
                                    CIP

For Kenneth Jernigan
A man unsurpassed in integrity, determination and vision

PREFACE

I wish to thank a number of people for their contributions to this book. Professor Gary Albrecht provided both encouragement and assistance. The use of an early draft of his recent book, *The Disability Business: Rehabilitation in America,* was particularly helpful. Several of my colleagues read parts of the manuscript and I frequently benefited from their suggestions. They include: Kenneth Benson, John Galliher, Darlaine Gardetto, Richard Hessler, James McCartney, Andrew Twaddle, and Ted Vaughan.

I wish to thank Corinne Kirchner and Mary Ellen Mulholland of the American Foundation for the Blind for their comments and assistance in locating hard to find material. The library staff at the American Foundation for the Blind and the Perkins School for the Blind were very helpful.

Felicia Beckmann read the entire manuscript and made many helpful suggestions. Rick Pfeiffer provided invaluable editorial assistance throughout the process. Phoebe Rastorfer suffered much as she patiently worked with me in preparing several drafts of the manuscript. Thanks also to Judy Manlove for her many editorial suggestions.

My wife, JoAn Vaughan, who teaches at Stephens College-Columbia, Missouri, contributed many helpful suggestions.

I also wish to thank the countless volunteers at Recording for the Blind, Inc. Their work has greatly enriched my life and my education.

The Graduate School of the University of Missouri-Columbia provided invaluable support in the form of a research grant.

CONTENTS

THE STRUGGLE OF BLIND PEOPLE
FOR SELF-DETERMINATION

Chapter 1

INTRODUCTION

This book is about the struggle of blind people for self-determination. It focuses on recurring areas of conflict between the visually handicapped and those who would rehabilitate and educate them. Finally, it argues for a different way of thinking about blindness and for regarding, as central, the views of blind people themselves.

There is nearly silence in the professional literature about the struggle for the empowerment of blind people. It is a dangerous topic that threatens some of the basic ideas underlying the claim to professional status of those who work to educate and rehabilitate the blind and visually impaired. None of us need be reminded that there are many who agree with me and who unceasingly work for the empowerment and self-determination of blind people. However, because this book focuses on points of contention, it is imbalanced. It bypasses the good works of those professionals, both blind and sighted, who have enriched the lives of so many others.

Blind people are as diverse as any other minority group in our society. Some of them will say that this book is much ado about nothing, especially those who join forces with some leaders of the professions that argue for the status quo. These individuals believe that the interests of blind people are best served when those in power are not questioned or challenged. For them, cooperation at any cost is preferable because it will yield the highest level of public support for programs intended to benefit blind people, thus themselves.

Point of View

This book does not claim to speak for all blind people. It speaks for what others and I call the organized blind—a social movement, now more than 50 years old, of blind people who work for self-determination, equal treatment and full participation in society. There are many organizations of blind people, many with benevolent purposes; they are not our subject. Instead, much of my material about blindness comes from

3

the National Federation of the Blind and its members, who with unbending will, have fought for self-determination.

Also, this book largely disregards issues related to those people who incur blindness in late life. Because this is the most rapidly growing group of people with limited vision, rehabilitation programs aimed at independent living receive increasing attention, and now a small amount of federal funding. Instead, this book focuses on the congenitally blind and adventitiously blind who since early or mid-life have been the traditional clients of the education and rehabilitation system.

My central tenet is that the behavior of blind people is not a product of blindness or the amount of residual vision, but of socialization. The reactions of parents, teachers, siblings, peers, the health professions, rehabilitation counselors and the general public have defined the lifestyles of blind people, and distinct patterns have emerged. Even though culture and level of economic development modify these patterns, unnecessary dependency is present when one examines the issue with a cross national and cross cultural perspective.

Many blind people live independent, self-reliant lives. They are employed, well educated, pay taxes, and participate fully in society. They have families, raise children, and from their point of view experience blindness as primarily an inconvenience. Other blind people live isolated lives frequently characterized by self-pity and negative self-images. They frequently live in homes where parents or other relatives provide assistance. They are seldom employed and participate little in society outside their immediate support group. They have accepted a tragic definition of their life situation. The lifestyles of blind and visually handicapped people who have become dependent on the welfare system reflect another pattern. In larger cities they frequently rely upon agencies for recreational and social activities. They receive income from Supplemental Security Income and various forms of disability payments. They have often received extensive rehabilitation and education services but have been unable to find employment at a level of remuneration adequate to compensate for lost welfare benefits.

As a sociologist, I am interested in patterns of education, patterns of rehabilitation service, patterns of socialization and patterns of ideas about blindness that, in large part, produce the three distinct lifestyles described above. I examine the economic interests of professional groups and the patterns of domination and subordination which find expression in the processes of education and rehabilitation. By focusing on areas of conflict between blind people and those who would benefit them, we have a sociologically useful vantage point for analyzing the elaborate practices that produce patterns of blindness.

Blind and visually impaired people are as diverse in their human qualities as the rest of the population. Even without blindness, some of them would doubtless not be successful in society. Like sighted individuals, many have been successful despite obstacles, some have become totally dependent on the welfare system and are content, and others have become resigned to the worst definitions of what it means to be blind in our society.

Although I am a sociologist, I am not a disinterested observer. At age sixteen, nearly forty years ago, I experienced vision loss which led to my first encounter with the rehabilitation system. The counselors and testers I met recommended that I consider going to college, and the rehabilitation services of West Virginia paid a part of that cost. For the next twenty-five years my education continued and my career as a sociologist developed. I gave little thought to blindness, except insofar as it was occasionally a personal nuisance to me. I experienced feelings ranging from annoyance, to humor, to anger when encountering discrimination relating to my blindness. In 1978, an acquaintance invited me to attend an annual meeting of the National Federation of the Blind. I was struck by the philosophy about blindness being expressed by many speakers, the rigor of the organization, and the commitment to share with the public a more positive view of blindness, to promote employment opportunities, and to oppose discrimination. For me, the five day meeting was an introduction into a dynamic social movement. I was sufficiently interested by this first encounter, not only because of my personal history, but also as a sociologist wanting to learn more.

Subsequently, I began to attend a local chapter in my home city and continued to attend state and national conventions. Consistently recurring themes were self-help, self reliance, competitive employment, quality education, participation in society as active citizens, challenging other blind people to become responsible for their own lives, seeking justice and equal treatment for blind people, and educating the public about blindness. The democracy apparent in the organization, the spirit of good will and mutual support, and the goals mentioned above seemed as American as apple pie.

Since social movements usually emerge as participants react to conditions they consider unjust, an essential aspect of every movement's dynamics is its continuous focus on the causal agents of unacceptable conditions. I was soon informed about the "enemies" of the movement—agencies, organizations, and the leadership of some professional groups which blocked the way to progress. Nevertheless, I have also involved myself, as a citizen and sociologist, in some of these organizations of professionals. There were occasionally efforts to enlist me into the groups that were opposed to consumer empowerment. In many settings the hostility to the organized blind movement was palpable. I began to observe that the tension was particularly concentrated in the established leadership of some agencies and professional organizations. The conflict often swirled around strong personalities on both sides. However, the conflict, which will be described throughout this book, is far too intense and widespread to be explained in terms of personalities and individual actors.

Ironically, the positive goals and attitudes of the consumer movement were the same goals usually voiced by rehabilitation and education professionals. Yet the professional literature has ignored the conflict. While vilification has occurred on both sides, much time and many economic resources have been wasted and the general public confused. Explaining the social sources of this conflict has guided my research on this issue. Although this book is about the socialization of blind people, parallels to other kinds of dependency creating benevolent activity are apparent. Unnecessary or extrinsic dependency of the elderly, the deaf, the developmentally disabled, the poor, and others has an economic and organizational basis similar to that of the blindness rehabilitation system.

Sources and Perspectives

The material in this book comes from many different sources. I have reviewed archival sources related to the early development of the occupations usually called "work for the blind." I have examined the consumer and professional literature related to developments in the United States and also reviewed material from England, Canada, China, and other countries for a cross-national and cross-cultural perspective. For the past six years I have been a participant observer in both consumer and professional organizations. I have served on advisory boards at the local, county, state, and national levels. For example, I am on the editorial board of the Journal of Visual Impairment and Blindness and have served on the advisory board for the Rehabilitation Services of Missouri. I serve as a Fair Hearing Officer for the Rehabilitation Services of

Missouri. Although never holding elected offices, I have been a regular participant of the National Federation of the Blind at the local, state, and national levels. I have formally interviewed more than one hundred people and informally interviewed hundreds more. I have visited and observed residential rehabilitation centers, including, for research purposes, a two week stay in a residential rehabilitation center. Finally, but not least in importance, I was a client of the vocational rehabilitation system. In addition to the interviews, participant observation, and historical research, I have attempted to consistently use concepts from sociology to help explain patterns of autonomous and heteronomous behavior which I have observed and which are frequently discussed in the literature. I focus on the point where conflict has emerged between consumers and professionals. I locate the source of the conflict in the economic and social advantages being protected from consumer empowerment.

This book is critical in its perspective. My purpose is to analyze patterns of domination and subordination which I and many other people judge harmful. I have no sympathy for social inequality based on gender, ethnicity or physical condition. Many blind people have had their lives unnecessarily restricted while, in the name of benevolence, others who are sighted have advanced in their careers, increased their social prestige, and gained control of economic resources. While none of these undesirable conditions occur everywhere in the blindness rehabilitation system, they occur frequently enough. By making the social and economic roots of conflict between consumers and the agencies where professionals are employed more explicit, I hope to contribute to a broader based and better informed dialogue. I hope some blind readers of this book will achieve fuller understanding and thus be able to deal better with some of the difficulties they are encountering as they seek assistance for education and employment. I also hope this book will make a small contribution to the redefinition of blindness on the part of some professional rehabilitation workers, some blind people, and some educators. This research should also be of interest to social scientists who are analyzing dependency in the modern welfare state. Finally, since much public money is spent on programs related to disability, this book should inform citizen understanding and related public policy debates.

The Plan of the Book

Chapter 2 develops the sociological perspective used in this book. I consistently use sociological concepts concerning bureaucracies, professions, social classes, minority groups, and political and economic power to explain patterns of domination and subordination which are analyzed throughout this book in different cultural and social contexts. There are multiple sources of human behavior and two of the most universal are the economic and social interests of groups of people, in this case, people in similar occupations. Ideas or ideals can be another source. The efforts of organizations of blind people for equal treatment have occurred in the context of the entire society, and the empowerment of blind people contributed to and was also augmented by the convergence of several movements for equal rights during the 1960s and 1970s.

Chapter 3 analyzes characteristics of the work setting where rehabilitation occurs. The rehabilitation industry is described and the major players in the blindness rehabilitation sector are reviewed. The consumer as both raw material and product is depicted. I conclude by describing the response of the organized blind movement to the bureaucratic domination of rehabilitation and education efforts.

In Chapter 4, I consider a major source of frustration to many blind and disabled persons; they think of themselves as ordinary people, but, they must continually deal with well-meaning people who, unfortunately, have acquired pervasive cultural stereotypes and images about blindness and blind people. This chapter analyzes the interaction process itself. In addition, it examines the special ideas professionals bring to the interaction with clients. These include the fundamental negative bias which results when researchers continually focus on an aspect they have defined as a problem, and paradigms about blindness such as those constructed to describe the relationship between visual perception and "reality" which appear throughout the professional literature. Changing what it means to be blind is the central issue in consumer responses to these stereotypes and to relationships dominated by citizens and professionals who hold negative images about blindness.

Chapter 5 elaborates upon one of the themes introduced in Chapter 4. Claims about being scientific and objective were soon followed by calls for professionalization. Using the "prestige" of science, a new terminology was created to describe special and severe problems caused by the absence of visual perception. Thus, professionals defined blindness as a traumatic condition with unique characteristics. Special intervention was required and it could only be provided by these experts. Their new ideas for the blindness system were touted as legitimate because they were based upon science and research. They were used to buttress professional claims. From the consumer point of view, most of these ideas were unnecessary and harmful both to the rehabilitation process and blind people themselves.

Chapter 6 then details the efforts of some professionals to coordinate and dominate the field of blindness rehabilitation. As a case study, this chapter examines the origins, development and recent history of a certification process which places its stamp of approval on compliant agencies. The issue over agency accreditation has resulted in the longest and bitterest battle—that between the National Federation of the Blind and the National Accreditation Council of Agencies Serving the Blind and Visually Handicapped. Consumer participation and the presumed threat to professional expertise and power are at the center of the struggle.

Chapter 7 focuses on professionals who function in formal bureaucratic settings. Also examined are the consequences of rehabilitation services when they become subordinated to organizational and professional interests. We look at the conflict which emerges when those served challenge the legitimacy of those purporting to serve. The historic rise of the profession is reviewed along with the resultant consumer resistance. Ultimately, the activities of members of the bureaucracy include the defense of vested interests by those having greater power, the social control and domination of subordinates by superordinates, the specialization of work and related claims of expertise, and a refined and developed rhetoric justifying the entire process.

Finally, in the last chapter I examine alternatives to many present approaches to rehabilitation and identify characteristics of what I consider to be particularly successful programs. Here we study organizational characteristics, the empowerment of blind people, and desirable philosophies of blindness.

In the first paragraph of this introduction I mentioned that we will take as a departure point the ideas of blind people themselves. At the conclusion of each chapter I present several relevant articles, letters, statements or other materials which have appeared in the consumer literature. Observing how blind people themselves see the issues being discussed is critical to understanding the conflict described in this book and to recognizing the aspirations of blind people. Although some of the statements are dated, the situations which evoke them continue to occur.

This book is about the struggle for equal treatment, dignity, and participation in society for blind people and their fellow travelers among the sighted. Since there are those who continue to regard blind people with negative stereotypes, the battle is far from over. Human resistance to domination, exploitation, dehumanization and arbitrary treatment is primal.

The story of Oliver Twist, although not about a blind person, demonstrates many of the issues discussed in this book. Oliver was a poor boy, a ward of the state, and a recipient of custodial treatment. He was continually subjected to arbitrary treatment by those assigned to care for him. His care included the most menial work and the most subordinate position in the household in which he was placed. Oliver's sense of dignity was sorely tried by those over him. In one instance his indignation sparked anger and even physical resistance. One of his caretakers, Mrs. Sowerberry, called in Mr. Bumble, an expert of the welfare system, to explain and deal with Oliver's recalcitrance.

> "It's not Madness, ma'am," replied Mr. Bumble, after a few moments of deep meditation. "It's Meat."
>
> "What?" exclaimed Mrs. Sowerberry.
>
> "Meat, ma'am, meat," replied Bumble, with stern emphasis. "You've overfed him, ma'am. You've raised a artificial soul and spirit in him, ma'am, unbecoming a person of his condition: as the Board, Mrs. Sowerberry, who are practical philosophers, will tell you. What have paupers to do with soul or spirit? It's quite enough that we let 'em have live bodies. If you had kept the boy on gruel, ma'am, this would never have happened." (Dickens, 1838/1990, p. 47)

Chapter 2

A SOCIAL PERSPECTIVE ON DEPENDENCY, CITIZEN EMPOWERMENT, AND HUMAN RIGHTS

Only in the past three decades have the social sciences focused much attention upon people with disabilities. Much energy has been directed into empirical studies of stereotypes and images of people with disabilities (Altman, 1981; Bogdan et al., 1982; Gartner, 1982; Longmore, 1985; Richardson et al., 1961). Albrecht (1981) analyzed the concept of disability as a social problem and described the early dominance of the medical model. It soon became apparent that definitions of disability by professionals involved subjective elements and reflected class interests, levels of technological development and cultural values. This awareness led to various forms of deviance models constructed to explain attitudes toward, and the treatment of, disabled persons (Albrecht, 1984; Sussman, 1969; Twaddle, 1973). The most widely cited sociological monographs were *The Making of Blind Men* (1969) by Robert Scott and *Stigma* (1961) by Erving Goffman.

All previous work has one common characteristic—the level of analysis is social-psychological. Hence, the focus has been on the individual, his or her attitudes, self-concepts, socialization, and interaction with professionals and others. Despite much consumer unrest and questions about the effectiveness of disability programs, little attention has been paid to the organizational context in which rehabilitation services occur. This chapter does not examine the individual blind person or rehabilitation worker, but the work setting and interest groups that control economic resources available for education and rehabilitation programs. In this chapter, I offer a sociological explanation of the conflict between the consumers of rehabilitation services and those who would educate and rehabilitate them. This conflict has stimulated the disability rights movement, which provides an excellent opportunity to see the world from its developing subculture perspective.

Economic Resources and Bureaucratic Structures

Weber (1978/1920) linked the growth of bureaucratic structure to the control of economic resources, which he thought to be central to the creation of wealth and power. Looking beyond production in the economic arena, he extended Marx's ideas to most institutional sectors of society. "The bureaucratic structure goes hand in hand with the concentration of material means of management in the hands of the master" (p. 980). Bureaucratic structures link not only capitalist enterprises, but those in the public sector as well. For example, of the bureaucratic structure of the modern army he said, "War in our time is a war of machines, and this makes centralized provisioning technically necessary, just as the dominance of the machine in industry promotes the concentration of the means of production and management" (p. 981). He similarly extended his historical analysis of the centralization of economic resources to higher education. His arguments now apply to all levels of education in the modern state. Researchers and teachers are separated from their means of production just as factory workers are separate from theirs. Standardization through bureaucratic control is a dominant feature of contemporary education.

Mass social movements in democracies demonstrate the same bureaucratizing process (p. 984). In extending his analysis to the modern welfare state, Weber found that patterns of economic influence and the degree of political domination vary with the size of the activity in question. Economic and other interests underlie social arrangements by which one group subordinates others. Holders of political and economic resources, including cultural transmission institutions, are the focus of our efforts to understand persistently enduring structures of relationships which alter the life chances of subordinate groups. Examining the resistance of subordinated groups can explain the mechanisms that perpetuate domination (Adam, 1978, p. 4).

In Chapter 3, I review the extent to which the rehabilitation industry has become big business. Then, throughout the remainder of this book, I show that political control of the rehabilitation process resides with interest groups located in bureaucratically organized work settings.

A rather sizeable body of literature exists with respect to organizational dimensions of client centered bureaucracies and their relations to agency policies, programs and practices. Scott (1969), for example, examined the network of organizations offering services to the blind and found that, among other consequences, certain features lead to the systematic displacement of agency goals. Constraints on financial resources and the imperative of efficiency have caused agencies to neglect programs which prepare clients for independent living in favor of those which can be measured in terms of money. In examining the relation of bureaucracy to the lower class, Sjoberg (1966) and his colleagues have argued that organizational features, such as the efficiency principle, convert welfare state agencies, established to assist lower class persons to break out of the "culture of poverty," into the single most important mechanism for maintaining and reinforcing patterns and conditions of lower class life. To ensure success, these agencies routinely funnel disproportionate amounts of resources to those clients already having the greatest likelihood of success. Lipsky (1980) has further noted that welfare state agencies possess characteristics that frustrate the best intentions of workers and demand either adjustments to the organization or withdrawal from it. These and numerous other examples point to the powerful implications of organizational structure upon those who provide services within these settings.

Bureaucratic patterns of domination are extremely resistant to change except insofar as change serves to solidify the power of bureaucratized social action. Critical or reflective opinions of the individual bureaucrat count for little. His or her very modes of thinking are linked to the position he occupies in the bureaucratic structure, which is linked to other hierarchically ordered positions. "For example, those in power are less constrained by the rules than those below. However, they also have a special interest in sustaining their privilege and thus their reflectivity is constrained by their commitment to 'system maintenance'" (T. Vaughan and Sjoberg 1993, p. 10). They cannot "squirm out of the apparatus" in which they are employed.

> Once fully established, bureaucracy is among those social structures which are the hardest to destroy. Bureaucracy is the means of transforming social action into rationally organized action. Therefore, as an instrument of rationally organizing authority relations, bureaucracy was and is a power instrument of the first order for one who controls the bureaucratic apparatus. (Weber, 1978/1920, p. 987)

Thus, democracy, in the sense of citizen influence with possibility of control is particularly at risk.

> We must expressly recall at this point that the political concept of democracy, deduced from "equal rights" of the governed, includes these further postulates:

(1) prevention of the development of a closed status group, and (2) minimiza-
tion of the authority of officialdom in the interest of expanding the sphere of
influence of "public opinion" as far as practicable. (Weber, 1978/1920, p. 985)

In his analysis of bureaucratic rationality, Weber was concerned with
the issues of personal responsibility, human freedom, and creativity; this
theme was also common to many early sociologists who observed the
consequences of rational bureaucratic forms of economic production in
the factory system. One of the contradictions between human rights and
rational bureaucratic forms of organization is that they occupy the same
social space.

> For Weber, freedom, creativity and personal responsibility did not lie outside
> the scope of society, of social relations and activities. On the contrary, interper-
> sonal relations, organizations, institutional structure and the macro-societal
> setting constituted the arena in which freedom, creativity, and responsibility
> are manifest. (Eisenstadt, 1968, p. xvi)

Dominant social characteristics, particularly rational bureaucracy,
impose severe limitations on freedom, frequently sufficient to create
alienation not only in the economic arena, but in all spheres of social organization. Weber perceived face-to-face relations, social groups and
organizations, and macro-social and cultural arrangements as massive
structural frameworks within which human beings enjoy but little freedom and few possibilities of change or development and exercise of
personal responsibility.

Accordingly, freedom and responsibility exist primarily in organized
settings and paradoxically arise from challenges to existing conditions.
Charismatic leaders emerge as they challenge present arrangements and
their followers sometimes become organized in social movements. One
approach is to attempt to change organizational patterns over time by
bringing external political influence to bear. Another approach is to
create alternative structures which minimize the conditions infringing
on human rights. Much of the remainder of this book describes the
conflict which has resulted from the clash between bureaucratic forms of
organization and the social movement which seeks the empowerment
of blind people.

Bureaucratic Patterns and the Delivery of Human Services

According to Weber (1978/1920), modern bureaucracy exhibits the
following characteristics: official jurisdiction determined by laws or administrative regulations, necessary duties regarded as official duties, and

employees having requisite qualifications. Coordination results in clear authority relationships—power is from the top down. For those who follow regulations, employment is relatively secure, which frequently constitutes a career. Employees are evaluated and organizational activities are documented and these records are preserved to permit accountability and judgments about organizational efficiency.

As Weber observed, rational bureaucratic forms of organization, which arose in the late Middle Ages in the West, came into being to counter capricious judgments made by officials who had inherited, purchased or otherwise obtained positions of power. In the modern bureaucratic pattern, laws and regulations are generally applied to individual cases. Thus, relationships at different levels of a bureaucracy including the human service sector, between employees and those seeking education, rehabilitation or other services are impersonal. Finally, the individual employed in the large organization is expected to demonstrate loyalty.

We now use the term "whistle blower" to describe former employees who upon departure expose alleged wrong-doings by their former employer. Being a "team player" is a minimal requirement for career advancement. Since loyalty includes protecting internal problems of the organization from outside scrutiny, secrecy becomes an organizational characteristic. As Weber (1978/1920) noted,

> Bureaucratic administration always tends to exclude the public, to hide its knowledge and action from criticism as well as it can. . . . This tendency towards secrecy is in certain administrative fields a consequence of their objective nature: namely, wherever power interests of the given structure of domination toward the outside are at stake, whether this be the case of economic competitors of a private enterprise or that of potentially hostile foreign politics in the public field. (p. 992)

Of course, annual reports present only the favorable side of an organization. As demonstrated many times in this book, the consumer movement of blind people has frequently exposed financial mismanagement, sexual and economic exploitation, and questionable educational and rehabilitation practices. Of necessity the information is obtained by "inside informants," "whistle blowers," and investigative journalists. Because of the internal hierarchical control of information, citizen or consumer access is difficult. "The concept of the 'office secret' is the specific invention of bureaucracy, and few things it defends so fanatically as this attitude which, outside of the specific areas mentioned, cannot be justified with purely functional arguments" (Weber, 1978/1920, p. 992).

Not to protect organizational interests and secrets may be extremely detrimental to an employee's future prospects. As representatives of the organized structure of power, social service personnel are paid laborers dependent upon the ongoing processes of the organization for their livelihood. For many of them there are almost no employment alternatives other than similar positions at other bureaucratic agencies.

Many rehabilitation workers may not have experienced competitive employment before entering the bureaucratically organized agency. Lack of work experience and narrowly defined work qualifications minimize alternatives and encourage them to firmly attach themselves to an agency and its related job security. Technical job specialization and long term career aspirations traditional to the bureaucratic setting often create conditions inimical to successful rehabilitation outcomes. According to Joyce Scanlan, Director of BLIND (Blindness: Learning in New Dimensions), Inc., Minneapolis, Minnesota, a client anticipates training or education appropriate to facilitate employment in the wider society, while the rehabilitation employee, whether blind or not, has frequently never experienced work outside the agency setting (personal communication, September 14, 1992). The service provider's own narrow training within the protected work environment results in a narrowed range of expectations for clients. Wags have referred to such settings as "sheltered workshops." Thus, one of the earliest, and hence most critical, "role models" a client encounters may reflect behavior and attitudes which make competitive employment in a wide array of occupations impossible.

To summarize, consumers of rehabilitation services often find that they have no power in relationships with a counselor or a teacher. The counselor or teacher has little or no control relative to that of supervisors or administrators. Consequently, there is a strong impetus, as Weber (1978/1920) noted, for agency personnel to become extensions of the inherent power arrangements. Specialization dictates that each worker deal with only one narrowly defined activity. Clients have no alternative except, occasionally, other similar organizations. Documentation methods, employee loyalty and patterns of secrecy make arbitrary treatment and exploitation difficult to confirm. Conditions inherent in bureaucracies sometimes cause clients to feel dehumanized and managed, and they do much to explain why the oft-stated goals of rehabilitation may seem quite remote from the ongoing operation.

Professionals in Bureaucracies

Another dimension of economic control and power in modern bureaucracies is the presence of professional workers. Conflict within the organization frequently results when high status and well established professions operate within a bureaucratic setting, such as physicians working in hospitals. This is generally not the case for lower status professions and those occupational groups in the early stages of the process of professionalization. For the latter, the organizational setting is usually an asset, both economically and for legitimization by association.

Lower status and newly developing professions normally attempt to establish legitimacy and recognition by the general public and other professions. The solo practitioner is now a rarity in the blindness rehabilitation industry. Organizational interests have not been an obstacle to development and seldom a source of conflict. Organizational task specialization and the division of labor within the agency are complemented by nascent professional aspirations. Through professionalization, expertise is institutionalized, knowledge is specialized and employment constitutes a career.

According to Abbott (1988), "We have professionalism, in the first place, because our market based occupational structure favors employment based on personally held resources, whether of knowledge or of wealth" (p. 324). The situation as described applies to almost all occupational groups claiming professionalization in the burgeoning service sector of our economy. A general knowledge base is claimed but the worker's direct intervention into the life of the consumer is thought essential. The knowledge base must be "uncommodifiable," and in providing service to humans, professional intervention is necessary. General rules or theories require specific interpretations, and professionalization has been applied to most human problems. "To speak, as some have done, of moral entrepreneurship is to unduly limit the capacity of professions; they seize all sorts of human activities, not just the moral ones" (p. 324). In most cases, professional activities are practiced directly or indirectly on others in areas such as education, social work, architecture, control of many types of deviant behavior, health, aging, and rehabilitation services.

Throughout this study I focus on the consequences of professional behavior for the student or client. I examine consumer response to the professional behavior of rehabilitation experts and find that the bureaucratically organized resource base in which most professionals work is the source of most conflicts. Professions are market based organizations attempting to dominate and define areas of social concern (Larson, 1977). The resources available in the large scale bureaucratic work setting can be withheld when knowledge claims are questioned by consumers. The rehabilitation profession expands its market by creating new claims and thus more effectively appealing to the public for recognition and financial support. For example, we now have rehabilitation engineers, parapatologists, and interior designers specializing in work site adaptation.

Since machines now enable unskilled labor to perform highly skilled tasks, the factory model for organizing work now typifies most professional work sites. A dominant characteristic of modern professional activity is the structure of the work setting. There are divisions of labor within professional groups and rehabilitation, and frequently related professional groups work in the same bureaucratic setting. In this setting, professional expertise comes to include the interpretation of laws and regulations. "Much current expertise resides in the rules of these and other organizations of professionals, most of which are either overtly heteronomous or governed by professionals more or less openly identified as professional administrators" (Abbott, 1988, p. 325). In the professionalization of "work for the blind," the agency or organizational work setting has been a particularly important resource. For example, practitioners interested in education and welfare issues affecting blind people created an organization with national scope to aid the development of the profession (see Chapter 6). The resulting American Foundation for the Blind has become one of the dominant organizations in this field in economic resources and numbers of professional employees. It attempts to coordinate activities with smaller agencies and the federal government to set agendas for new developments.

To summarize, the field of "work for the blind" is undergoing professionalization. Creating organizations and intellectual claims has been an ongoing process in the United States for the last fifty years. Because claims are not always recognized by consumers of services or other competing professional groups, large scale organizations have grown to strengthen the power base of relatively weak "workers for the blind." As a result, large agencies and publicly funded state programs frequently represent the only economic resources available to blind people seeking rehabilitation services. Even if the consumer dismisses the claims of professionals, he or she may look the other way in order to obtain desired resources. These resources thus give more control to professionals in this field, and are also used to defend nascent professions from other competing or better established groups. The organizational work settings include the many branches of both federal and state government that provide educational, rehabilitation, and support programs, schools for the blind, university training centers, and hundreds of private agencies and sheltered workshops. These are linked by a social network reinforced by frequent regional and national conferences, journals, newsletters and social networks for employment opportunities.

Professionals and Consumer Empowerment

Our focus is on professionals who work in highly organized occupational settings, most frequently with an individual client or student. Equally important is the interaction between professional groups and consumer organizations. Here leaders of both haggle over policy, accountability, and consumer involvement in the rehabilitation process. As later chapters demonstrate, intense conflict occurs in both contexts and for similar reasons.

The profession interacts with the consumer in three major ways. First, status distinctions within the profession lead to indifferent responses to consumer challenges. Higher status, usually reflected by greater specialization, greater longevity in the profession and higher position within the organization, allows for infrequent interaction with the consumer. Thus, the newer, less specialized and less powerful worker interacts more often with clients. Any internal professional or organizational conflict resulting from consumer questions will be filtered through lower level workers and resolved by articulations from those of higher status. I have often encountered individual professionals who are frequently unwilling to discuss controversial issues with consumers—particularly at conferences or other gatherings where other professionals are present. Rhetoric and policy decisions are managed by those most removed from consumer concerns. In one recent discussion of accountability and program related issues, an agency administrator told the group of professionals that her highest priority was to preserve her agency (J. Scanlan, personal communication, September 14, 1992). Unfortunately, such statements are not surprising. However, in the presence of other professionals and consumers, such priorities are usually buried under several layers of traditional statements of professional goals and values. Such statements are a clear reflection of the industrial model operating within the rehabilitation industry. If the firm fails, everything of economic importance to the worker is gone.

> Since professionals draw their self-esteem more from their own world than from the public's, this status mechanism gradually withdraws entire professions into the purity of their own worlds. The front line service that is both their fundamental task and their basis for legitimacy becomes the province of low-status colleagues and para-professionals. (Abbott, 1988, p. 119)

Second, lower status professionals are threatened by rising levels of education among consumers who more and more question the knowledge base. Issues in rehabilitation are of obvious interest to blind people seeking such services and the more reflective among them may frequently be fully aware of and sensitive to them. When interacting with such consumers, the lower status professional's defense is to resort to the opinions, research, and status of professional elites. This includes appeals to models of blindness (see Chapter 5) which demonstrate that any blind person is, in principle, deficient. For example, the past two decades have witnessed the efforts of the largest professional organization, the Association for the Education and Rehabilitation of the Blind and Visually Impaired, to impose a vision requirement for those who want to teach mobility to blind people (see Chapter 7). Informed blind consumers generally reject this position as being discriminatory, uninformed, and featherbedding, while the professional considers it an issue of safety. Also, the licensed professional possesses something even the best informed blind client lacks—vision. Regardless of how the consumer views them, they control the organization based resources needed by the client. "In effect," he or she draws "upon organizational power as well as the power of his expertise to control the circumstances under which service is given" (Haug and Sussman, 1969, p. 155). I have observed, as has Larson (1977), that consumer questioning sometimes evokes anger from professionals.

> [H]ostility toward the client may be the norm. This manifests itself, ordinarily, in interpersonal contacts: the professional demands deference and compliance, denies any active participation in the process to the client, and enforces maximum social distance. Such hostility appears to be common among professionals who are themselves subordinate, and therefore insecure of their status, when forced to deal with lower-class clienteles. (p. 188)

Third, it is in the interest of professionals, particularly those working in institutional settings, to depoliticize consumers. Clients must not have any power within the organization because such power is contrary not only to professional ideologies about client limitations and professional knowledge, but also to patterns of organizational control. Organizations of professionals may, without much danger, co-opt individual consumers — being "in the presence of power" and other small perquisites may be sufficient reward (see Chapter 8). They have no power and can easily be isolated. Representatives of consumer organizations regularly encounter agency professionals who resist the idea that democratically elected leaders can speak for other consumers. However, it is far easier to run off an individual than the elected representative of a larger organization.

The National Federation of the Blind has consistently pointed out that it is an organization *of* the Blind, and, that its elected leaders can speak *for* the blind. For the Federation, consumer representation means more than tokenism, both numerically and philosophically. This stance is prima facia at odds with organizational and professional interests, and a conflict results (see Chapters 6, 7, and 8).

> It is a distinctive characteristic of the technobureaucratic ideology that it should make depoliticization of the citizenry into a major connotation of the "rule by experts." Ideological appeals to the safeguard of professional judgments and professional integrity can be used by all professions when they are threatened with client revolt or, more mildly, with client demands for some rights of review. Technobureaucratic professions participate fully in this ideological practice. It is unthinkable, however, that professionals whose power *depends* on hierarchy and on the bureaucratic uses of secrecy should ever invite clients to share in the organizational power. (Larson, 1977, p. 189)

The tendencies of bureaucratic rationality, which are further reinforced by professionals working in organizational settings, do more than frustrate and anger consumers. They also produce patterns of domination which threaten the autonomy, responsibility and creativity of individuals. The response has been an attempt to clarify the concept of human rights and to understand and correct social arrangements which limit them.

Human Rights and Their Implementation

As we noted, Weber was concerned about the effects of bureaucratic forms of social organization on human freedom and creativity. Human rights now dominate political rhetoric in many parts of the world, including the United Nations and many individual nation states. Amnesty International and other organizations monitor the denial of human rights in many countries. Violations of civil rights are continually decried, recent examples being the widespread public response to the Rodney King beating by police in Los Angeles and questions raised during the disintegration of Yugoslavia.

More generally, some social theorists and sociologists have focused upon the unity or similarity of conditions that result in human misery or suffering. As Barrington Moore (1966) has observed, humans do not like to be treated arbitrarily or have their safety and security or that of their families threatened. Many observers have noted that the historic intent of English Common Law was to extend equal treatment through the legal process to successively less powerful citizens.

More recently, researchers have focused on a conceptual clarification of human rights. Walter (1984, p. 430) claims that human rights include autonomy and self-esteem—seeing a purpose in life, not being used by others solely to promote their ends, having some control over one's life, and having some level of competence that aids in this control.

In *Taking Rights Seriously* (1977), Dworkin examines arguments underlying the concept of human rights from a particular theoretical perspective within the legal tradition. He notes that there are ways of treating people that are inconsistent with recognizing them as full members of the human community. However, weaker members of a political community are entitled to the same concern and respect from their government as are the more powerful members. All should be treated as human beings who have feelings, frustrations, and aspirations, and all should be treated as having the capacity for intelligent self determination.

While considering abstract or general philosophic ideas about human freedom, Bauman (1988) grounds his analysis in a social context.

> In the magnificent legacy the founders of sociology left us, "freedom" appears relatively seldom. In the main body of social theory, serious considerations of the "social conditioning" of freedom are few, far between and marginal. On the other hand, there is a lot of interest in, and profound observations about "social constraints," pressures, influences, power, coercion and whatever other man-made factors were blamed for preventing freedom, that natural endowment of every human being, from manifesting itself. (p. 4)

In the period leading up to the Industrial Revolution, especially in England and Holland, the concept of freedom became linked to the emerging economic system, best summarized in Adam Smith's *Wealth of Nations* (1976/1776). The capitalist market place was characterized as one in which each person made free choices. The economy would most flourish when individuals were least constrained. This new economic philosophy, linked with new technological developments, resulted in the Industrial Revolution. The freedom of some led to great wealth and power which shaped social conditions that denied choice to others and led to new patterns of poverty and domination. For a thorough analysis of the relationship between human rights, civil society and the state see "Civil Society and Social Theory," by Andrew Arato and Jean Cohen.

Separating the concept of individual freedom from that of morality in the social order has become the subject of much political and economic discourse. To base this on Adam Smith is to take one section of his work out of its broader context (Wolfe, 1989).

> But the market as a metaphor for a process of exchange that would serve as a moral model for all of society's interaction would have been a foreign idea to Adam Smith. In *a* market, friends can rely on their knowledge of one another and the trust they have developed to smooth over economic transaction. But in *the* market, friends are forced to treat one another as potential impediments to self-interest. If we organize all our social relations by the same logic we use in seeking a good bargain, we cannot even have friends, for everyone else interferes with our ability to calculate conditions that will maximize our self-interest. Take away the paradox that was clear to Adam Smith and one takes away what, to Smith, was one of the greatest sources of progress in the modern world: a private space in which authenticity and individuality could flourish. It is not simply that Adam Smith never thought to extend the principle of self-interest to all social relations; on the contrary, Smith recognized that to do so would destroy the very realm of morality that made economic self-interest possible in the first place. (p. 30)

Adam Smith's earlier and related work, *The Theory of Moral Sentiments* (1976/1759), is usually ignored by contemporary apologists for unconstrained capitalism.

As noted earlier, economic production was associated with new forms for organizing work. The factory system was extended through bureaucratic rationality to all arenas of society. In client-centered bureaucracies the recipients of services become commodities, are subordinate and have little freedom. The opposite is the case for those who dominate and control such organizations.

How are human rights to be preserved in societies dominated by bureaucratic rationality? How can subordinate people exercise choice? Pervasive patterns of bureaucratic organization are not likely to go away. Can the social sciences suggest alternative models of organization which will have fewer harmful consequences for those in subordinate positions? (See Chapter 8.) Finally, under what conditions can empowerment occur?

Human Rights through Democratic Association

John Dewey (1920) linked the intelligent behavior of the individual to social interaction with others. When we talk abstractly about the state, bureaucracy, or human rights rather than this or that group of suffering human beings, or this or that social arrangement, it is frequently easy to detract attention from specific problems (p. 188–190). For example, "Although Hegel asserted in explicit form that the end of states and institutions is to further the realization of freedom of all, his effect was to consecrate the Prussian State and to enshrine bureaucratic absolutism" (p. 190). Accordingly, there is a tendency to minimize the importance of specific conflicts. "Since in theory the individual and the state are reciprocally necessary and helpful to one another, why pay much attention to the fact that in this state a whole group of individuals are suffering from oppressive conditions?" (p. 191) Without a different approach, as Dewey noted, we are thrown back on short sighted opportunism, crude empiricism or the "matching of brute forces" (p. 192). Problems are dealt with by citing precedence, attempting conciliation or adjustment, or using coercive force (p. 192).

While Dewey examined the primacy of individuality in communication, our focus is on the impact of economic and social arrangements on interacting individuals. "Is the capacity which is set free also directed in some coherent way, so that it becomes a power, or its manifestations spasmodic and capricious?" (p. 197) Inquiries must always be specific. Are our sensibilities heightened or dulled by this or that form of organization?

> Like utilitarianism, the theory subjects every form of organization to continual scrutiny and criticism. But instead of leading us to ask what it does in the way of causing pains and pleasures to individuals already in existence, it inquires what is done to release specific capacities and coordinate them into working powers. (p. 198)

These capacities become linked through association as individuals communicate with each other about common values.

More recently, Wolfe (1989) has analyzed the issue of moral agency, in a manner consistent with Dewey.

> In the sociological tradition—and even then only in that part which rejects an emphasis on social structure in favor of the notion that ordinary people

create moral rules through everyday interaction with others—lies an understanding of moral agency that allows us to bring people back in to modernity,
to begin to give them the control in the making of moral rules that the market
and the state promised but never delivered. (p. 22)

Accordingly, association presumes equality—that individuals communicate when mutual respect characterizes interaction. Consumer empowerment is rooted in this understanding. General principals or understanding
created by "more superior" people cannot be an adequate basis of association because every person capable of association contributes to ongoing
developments. They are not passive recipients, broken vessels to be
mended, but other humans with a possibility of contributing to the
resolution of problems. When these individuals need to create additional forms of association a social movement or new organization becomes
a next step in the ongoing definition process.

> The increasing acknowledgement that goods exist and endure only through
> being communicated and that association is the means of conjoint sharing
> lies back of the modern sense of humanity and democracy. It is the saving
> salt in altruism and philanthropy, which without this factor degenerate
> into moral condescension and moral interference, taking the form of trying
> to regulate the affairs of others under the guise of doing them good or
> of conferring upon them some right as if it were a gift of charity. It follows
> that organization is never an end in itself. It is a means of promoting *associa-
> tion*, of multiplying effective points of contact between persons, directing
> their intercourse into the modes of greatest fruitfulness. (Dewey, pp. 206–
> 207)

A New Basis for Democratic Association

One consequence of the rehabilitation industry and of its predecessors,
welfare and educational institutions, was to bring individual blind people
together. Gradually, the educational level grew and blind people began
to be employed in a wide array of occupations. Some of them, through
their organizations, began to define themselves as a minority group
(Altman, 1981). I document this process throughout the remainder of the
book.

One result was that many individuals observed common patterns of
exploitation and subordination. They began to organize their own groups
and to educate their fellows about the social, educational and welfare
arrangements that had become, however well intended, barriers to their
maximal participation in society. Reflective blind people began to reject
the medical model of disability which located the "problem" within the

individual. As I note in Chapter 3, physicians and others associated with the medical industry are the gatekeepers of the rehabilitation process, for their diagnoses legitimate access to programs. Little attention is paid to the fact that the negative opinions of these professionals and others in the rehabilitation industry have been a primary source of consumers' difficulties. The medical and deviance models define human beings in terms of what no one wants to be.

> Hence neither is there any mention of the unfavorable attitudes that have made disabled women and men a deprived and disadvantaged minority facing one of the highest rates of unemployment and welfare dependency as well as a pattern of segregation in education, transportation, housing, and public accommodation that parallels the practice of apartheid. (Hahn, 1990, p. 104)

Opposition to these negative ideas has become a dominant concern of reflective blind people.

One aspect of this opposition is the development of positive alternative images which have strong implications for consumer involvement in the rehabilitation process. For example, the frequent focus on prevention, including the currently popular genetic engineering which would eliminate undesirable physical limitations, is called into question for suggesting the futile hope that such "bad" conditions may someday be gone. This elimination will not occur with the sort of intervention made by Hitler's doctors in the Third Reich, but with newer, more technologically sophisticated efforts. Rather than thinking exclusively of the elimination of disabilities, men and women may choose alternative approaches by which to identify with their "brothers and sisters" as a source of pride and dignity. "Black is Beautiful" was an important part of social revolution in the decade of the 1960s. Similar ideas abound in the blindness community where life with visual limitation may be viewed without negative feelings. The difficulties presented by physical characteristics may become a source of creativity, which may induce involvement in a social movement to help clarify human rights.

Having incorporated positive images in the social movement, members of the organized blind community seek to share their positive philosophy with the newly blinded or new generations of blind people. As mentioned earlier in this chapter, the position of many professionals is threatened by new and positive ideas about blindness. Their lack of knowledge further perpetuates dependency when they fail to direct their students and clients to associations with positive ideals and successful role models. The creation of new ideas and their introduction into the rehabilitation process is an example of how intelligent behavior can, through association, have influence on existing patterns of domination. Communities emerge reflecting new values and a subculture develops.

The blindness community is not a linguistic based subculture as is the deaf community. However, similar problems have been encountered. Just as blind people have been excluded from some occupations within the rehabilitation field, deaf people have also been excluded. Commenting on the treatment of the deaf community Lane (1992) writes:

> Paternalism's ignorance, I have explained, is self-serving. It is designed to reassure benefactors of the rightness of what they are doing, to protect them from the need for change, and to protect their economic interests. If the profession of deaf education acknowledged that deaf children have a language and that manual language is the best way to educate these children, then deaf adults would once again enter the profession (as they did in the last century), and hearing people would lose their monopoly. Paternalism and money are inseparable. (p. 38)

Partly as a result of the National Federation of the Blind's challenges to paternalistic treatment for more than fifty years, elements of a subculture have developed. A cultural heritage and a sense of generational continuity is developing. For example, Braille and the white cane are not simply symbols of this minority group, they are among its most cherished and positive tools for autonomy. This group produces its own books and journals at the national level and in almost every state. There is much loyalty to, dedication to, and respect for the leadership of the movement. The group takes pride in its values and consistently resists appropriation by broader based social movements or well funded agencies.

In accord with Dewey's ideas on democratic association, I maintain that the organized blind movement was a necessary social and economic response to existing patterns of domination. A disabling environment, arranged by educators and service providers, places unnecessary restrictions on different types of ability.

> The minority group perspective is predicated on the belief that prejudicial attitudes can be altered primarily through modification of institutions and behavior to facilitate equal status contacts between disadvantaged and dominate portions of society. (Hahn, 1990, p. 104)

Inequality of this type is remedied by political and legal action as well as public education and many forms of consumer pressure on agencies.

Interest groups will give up their advantages when it becomes advantageous to change. Continual efforts to re-educate such groups may help.

However, threats to funding sources and to claims of legitimacy are sometimes effective in quickening the pace of change. To this end, the social movement of the organized blind has power and is using it. First, it can withhold cooperation—if the intended beneficiaries of public and philanthropic programs decline to participate and publicly question the value of these programs, the involved agencies have a serious problem on their hands. Second, it has considerable economic resources contributed by its membership (see Chapter 3), which can be used to educate the public and politicians about the programs being questioned. Power will increase from effective nationwide organization for political lobbying and the willingness of the membership to demonstrate, picket, and pursue legislation to change policies and programs. The organized blind will continue to gain in influence and, as more professionals and service providers join in this social movement, spread the movement's philosophy throughout existing agencies.

This empowerment is based on the understanding of the value of the individual, corresponding commitments to human rights, patterns of association to challenge others to be reflective about their situation and the resulting democratic processes to move toward the movement's goals. The emerging social movement is challenged to create new forms of organization and association which can modify and even replace existing forms (see Chapter 8).

In the United States the Progressive era witnessed the application of large scale public efforts to solve social problems. If you are helping people, if you are doing them good, the more power the better. Quasi-legal regulations and programs gave overwhelming power to the newly developing occupation of social work and related occupations. The following article (Vaughan, 1990) describes these developments and consumer responses.

WHAT WENT WRONG WITH DOING GOOD

Many of us have observed defensive, caustic, and even angry behavior displayed by some professionals and some agency personnel when confronted with consumer criticism or demands for increased consumer participation. Critics are frequently dismissed as misguided and are certainly ungrateful for the contributions rehabilitation efforts have made in the lives of blind people. With so many professional organizations of workers for the blind, special programs informed by scientific research and continual support from government and the public, how could anyone question the beneficence of these efforts? Isn't "doing good" always desirable? How can beneficence be mischievous or even harmful?

David Rothman, a social historian at Columbia University, analyzes social programs that developed in the Progressive era in this country. Beginning around 1900, public energy and money was organized to deal with a wide array of social problems. "In the history of American attitudes and practices toward the dependent, no group more energetically or consistently attempted to translate the biological model of the caring parent into a program for social action than the Progressives" (Rothman, 1978, p. 69). We will utilize his idea of benevolence as disguised power and draw examples from his analysis of several welfare programs to clarify why many consumers resist efforts by those who would do them good.

In the first two decades of this century, the needs of the poor and dependent were widely noted. As Rothman observes, the state as parent had much to accomplish. Everyone would benefit. There was presumed unity of interests between the state and the several different types of needy citizens.

Agents of the welfare state were so committed to a paternalistic model that they never concerned themselves with the potential of their programs to be as coercive as they were liberating. "In their eagerness to play parent to the child, they did not pause to ask whether the dependent had to be protected against their own well-meaning interventions. It was as if the benevolence of their motives together with their clear recognition of the wretchedness of lower-class social conditions guaranteed that ameliorative efforts would unambiguously benefit the poor" (Rothman, p. 72).

As Rothman notes, there was consensus around the values of scholars and reformers alike. Schools, settlement houses, and a wide array of social programs would bring the poor and immigrants into the mainstream of middle-class American life. Between 1900 and 1920 many of our contemporary social welfare programs had their origins, including child support, juvenile courts, and, we might add, new and expanded programs to benefit blind people. The American Association of Workers for the Blind (AAWB) was organized in 1905 with a broad agenda which included employment, the welfare of elderly blind persons, boarding homes and other housing arrangements for blind adults, nurseries for blind babies, home teaching services for adults, and industrial education. The AAWB and the American Association of Instructors of the Blind (AAIB) grew, both in size and mutual concerns, and by 1921, jointly created the American Foundation for the Blind (AFB) as a new national resource for advancing their concerns.

What went wrong with the well-intentioned efforts of reformers to improve the lot of the poor, the widowed, the delinquent, the untutored immigrant, and the disabled? Since the aim of the state was to help the disadvantaged, there was no need to limit the power utilized for doing good.

In each instance, therefore, enabling legislation and agency practice enhanced the prerogatives of state officials—legal protections and rights for those coming under their authority. To call the acts "widow pensions" was really a misnomer. The widows did not receive their allowance as a matter of right, the way a pensioner received his. Rather, the widow had to apply for her stipend, demonstrate her qualifications, her economic need, and her moral worth, and then trust to the decision of the welfare board. At their pleasure, and by their reckoning, she then obtained or did not obtain help. By the same token the juvenile court proceedings gave no standing to the whole panoply of rights that offenders typically enjoyed, from a trial by jury to assistance from counsel, to protections against self-incrimination. There was nothing atypical about the juvenile court judge who openly admitted that in his Minnesota courtroom "the laws of evidence are sometimes forgotten or overlooked." So, too, probation officers were not bound by any of the restrictions that might fetter the work of police officers. They did not need a search warrant to enter a probationer's home, for as another juvenile court judge explained: "With the great right arm and force of the law, the probation officer can go into the home and demand to know the cause of the dependency or the delinquency of a child. . . . He becomes practically a member of the family and teaches them lessons of cleanliness and decency, of truth and integrity." So caught up were reformers with this image of officer as family member that they gave no heed to the coercive character of their programs. To the contrary, they frankly declared that "threats may be necessary in some instances to enforce the learning of the lessons that he teaches, but whether by threats or cajolery, by appealing to their fear of the law or by rousing the ambition that lies latent in each human soul, he teaches the lesson and transforms the entire family into individuals which the state need never again hesitate to own as citizens." With the state eager and able to accomplish so beneficent a goal, there appeared to no reason to restrict its actions.

The prevalence of such judgments among Progressives partially blinded them to the realities that followed on the enactment of their proposals. Not only did they fail to see the many inadequacies that quickly emerged in day-to-day operations, worse yet, they could not begin to understand that the programs might be administered in the best interests of officials, not clients. (Rothman, pp. 78–79)

One might say about many administrators of these programs that whatever else they did, they looked after the interests of their agencies and careers. Commenting on the history of original missionary families in Hawaii, comedians have observed, they came to do good and ended up doing well. We now observe widespread cynicism about the claims of self-appointed caregivers. Do-gooders are suspect. To quote Rothman again, "Whereas once historians and policy analysts were prone to label some movements reforms, thereby assuming their humanitarian aspects, they are presently far more comfortable with a designation of social control, thereby assuming their coercive quality" (p. 81).

Power and social control operate, in part, through organizational procedures and administrative discretion. We live in an age of regulations. countless agency conferences are held to "interpret the regs." Administrators and their subordinates control resources and apply rules. Clients, patients, or students have few alternatives. Power relationships are one-sided. Even our government has recognized this condition by funding protection and advocacy programs to give independent legal assistance and other support to individuals challenging their treatment at the hands of the rehabilitation system. Fair hearing officers are now used to hear client appeals in several states. We have an acute distrust of discretionary authority.

With the civil rights movement of the 1960s Rothman describes a trend evidenced in several different branches of the welfare rights movement. "The perspective is not the perspective of common welfare but the needs of the particular group. The intellectual premises are not unity but conflict. It is 'us' versus 'them' " (p. 90). Control and benevolent oversight have been self-consciously rejected and replaced with concerns about autonomy and civil rights. Do not deprive us of competitive employment, equal pay for equal work, opportunities for economic mobility because we are women, black, needing some medical intervention, poor, or perhaps, blind. Rehabilitation or other programs that block freedom of choice, from the perspective of this liberty and human rights concern, must be removed and are, indeed, not solutions but parts of the problem.

Expanding the liberty perspective, as Rothman notes, will not solve all of the problems of various minority interest groups. Legitimate needs remain. Appropriate education and opportunities for competitive employment are still essential elements of equal opportunity for blind people. Our concern, obviously, is not to promote neglect or legitimate cruelty and suffering in the name of rights. How can we access opportunities and utilize the resources of publicly funded programs and yet avoid domineering, demeaning, dependency-creating relationships with agents of rehabilitation? How can the power imbalance be redressed? Can we avoid throwing away the baby with the bath water? How can we limit discretionary and arbitrary authority associated with publicly supported programs?

"To this end, advocates of the liberty model are far more comfortable with an adversarial approach, an open admission of conflict of interest, than with an equality model with its presumption of harmony of interests" (p. 92). Would this human rights, liberty model be compatible with service and educational arrangements provided by experts, professionals, and public officials?

Whenever publicly supported programs are needed, the recipients of benevolence must have a determinative voice in policy making and evaluation. If you will do good to me, it will have to be on my terms—or we will, at least, have to be in agreement and with mutual respect. Being a determinative voice means full consumer participation. Such participation will not come from agency-selected individuals or self-appointed guardians of blind people, but from broadly-based, democratically elected representatives of organizations of blind people. (p. 362–365)

Organized services for blind people continue to expand. Bureaucracies develop new service programs. For example, most major universities now have access offices which provide services for students with disabilities. Staff at such offices provide services for blind students that could be done by the students themselves. If students did not have these special services they would interact more frequently with their instructors and acquire skills useful in other settings. In the following article which appeared in the *Braille Monitor* in October, 1992, Curtis Chong analyses the consequences of such services.

THE PITFALLS OF COMPLACENCY

From the Associate Editor: Curtis Chong is the Vice President of the National Federation of the Blind of Minnesota and President of the National Federation of the Blind in Computer Science, the computer science division of the National Federation of the Blind. His experience with disabled student services offices is unfortunately not uncommon. In the Spring, 1992, issue of "The Student Slate," the publication of the National Association of Blind Students, he wrote of his experience and warned his readers of the pitfalls that can befall those who rely unquestioningly on the services of disabled students offices. Here is what he has to say:

Many years ago, when I first began attending the University of Hawaii, I came across a program called Kokua. *Kokua* is a Hawaiian word meaning "help." The espoused purpose of the Kokua program was to help handicapped students attending the University of Hawaii; and, since I was blind, I was eligible to receive the help offered by the program.

Kokua maintained a staff of college students who served variously as readers, note takers, and guides. They were paid with rehabilitation funds. Kokua staff, for example, would perform the tedious and frustrating tasks involved in registration. Instead of having to stand in line for hours in a large and crowded gymnasium to register, blind students had merely to provide the helpful Kokua staff with the list of classes they wanted to take, and presto! they were registered.

Much of the time of the Kokua student staff was used recording college textbooks. The service was so efficient that blind students never had to find out during the previous semester what texts were going to be used for the current semester; Kokua had enough student readers available to tape books on demand.

Most blind students at the University of Hawaii loved the Kokua program. It did everything for them. They didn't have to plan ahead to have books taped. They never had to hire their own readers. They didn't have to stand in long registration lines. When tests needed to be taken, everything was handled by Kokua. Blind students didn't even have to learn how to travel independently; there was always a guide available to take them from class to class.

In short, blind students at the University of Hawaii became complacent, taking the services they received for granted. Perhaps even more tragic, many of them failed to recognize that their complacency was ruining their long-term prospects of a successful and productive future.

Consider the hiring of readers. The students employed by the Kokua program were paid for with rehabilitation funds. In fact, by the time I began attending the University of Hawaii, blind students were expressly prohibited from using rehabilitation funds to pay for their own personal readers. They were required to use the services of the Kokua staff. Thus, they were deprived of the invaluable experience of seeking out, hiring, supervising, and occasionally firing personal readers.

Many blind students never learned to be independent travelers, preferring instead to depend upon the helpful guides furnished to them by Kokua. Never venturing into unfamiliar territory on their own, they necessarily limited their prospects for future employment.

Each and every blind student on the University of Hawaii campus was regarded as a non-entity by most of the professors on campus. When a question came up about how a blind student would take a test, professors would invariably consult with the Kokua office rather than with the blind student. In fact, the Kokua staff members, not blind students, were consulted concerning all problems on campus involving blindness.

There were a few blind students on the University of Hawaii campus, including me, who recognized the existence of the problem and tried to deal with it. The system was, however, deeply entrenched, and our efforts were hampered by the fact that we were working in opposition to the basic desires of the many blind students who wanted to have things as easy as possible. Nevertheless, we did manage to achieve a small measure of success. We were able to establish a study area for blind students in one of the university's libraries, independent of the Kokua office. This allowed blind students to study on campus after Kokua staff locked up at 5:00 p.m. Additionally, we were able to prevail upon the state rehabilitation agency for the blind to permit rehabilitation funds to be used to pay for readers hired by individual blind students.

Back when I first started going to college, programs like Kokua were in the minority. Today, just about every major college campus in the country has some form of office specifically designed for students with disabilities. Some are more positive than others. It is human nature to take the easy way out and to let such offices do everything: recruit and hire readers, guide students from class to class, determine how tests will be taken, and provide staff to accomplish the tedious activities of course registration. Now as never before, blind students cannot afford to be complacent. For if they rely upon disabled student offices to handle even the most rudimentary aspects of their education, they will be selling themselves short and denying their tremendous potential to achieve true equality with their sighted peers.

If you are attending a college or university with an office for disabled students, ask yourself whether or not it is providing its services in a manner calculated to promote true independence. Is it encouraging students to gain invaluable expertise in the management of sighted readers? Are students expected to travel about campus independently? Are college professors encouraged to deal directly with the blind students in their classes instead of going to the office for disabled students? Are blind students expected to handle registration activities for themselves? If these questions cannot be answered in the affirmative, blind students must take immediate action to correct the situation.

Blind students cannot afford to permit complacency and the natural desire to take the easy way out to bolster an environment which encourages dependence, laziness, and irresponsibility. In today's corporate world there are no special services available to blind employees. Although my employer, IDS Financial Services, chose to purchase some assistive technology for me once I proved I could do the job of systems programming, company officials would laugh at the suggestion that a staff of readers and guides be made available to a blind employee. I am expected to travel anywhere to obtain technical training, and I am expected to manage my own sighted readers. IDS is not unique in this regard.

It is vitally important for college students to develop basic skills in independent travel, management of readers, and execution of their own college affairs; and it is critical that these skills be learned before or during college. Failure to develop these skills at the right time can and often does result in the loss of a paying job. (pp. 542–544)

Chapter 3

REHABILITATION AS BIG BUSINESS

In this book I examine the dependency which is unnecessarily created by programs and professionals intending to benefit persons with disabilities. I also focus on the conflict which sometimes results from interaction between clients and those who would rehabilitate them. A central argument of this book is that dependency and conflict, at least in part, arise from the work setting of those who provide rehabilitation services. Rehabilitation services have become a major growth industry in the United States, which involves much money, large organizations, many professional employees, and much specialized equipment. Management concerns about efficiency, cost containment, task specialization, specific regulations, and fiscal accountability have come to rule this work environment. In this chapter I identify the major characteristics of this industry, analyze the rehabilitation of blind people as a specialized sector of this industry, and discuss consumers' responses as they encounter the industry.

The Rehabilitation Industry

Increasing numbers of Americans are requiring rehabilitation due to accidents, work related chronic illnesses, following surgery or other medical interventions, or because of other conditions which prevent them from returning to or entering the labor force. Whether it be rehabilitation for physical or mental conditions or vocational rehabilitation leading to an individual's first efforts to enter the labor market, admission to this process is governed by physicians. The health industry is the major player, although special education and social welfare programs are also important. Rehabilitation programs are administered at the federal level under the Department of Health, Education and Welfare, while disability programs are administered under the Department of Health and Human Services.

For seventy years there has been a consistently high level of legislative support and funding for rehabilitation programs. As legislation has evolved, budget allocations have increased and, as Gary Albrecht has shown in his recent book *The Disability Business* (1992), now provide a major portion of the economic base for the rehabilitation business in the United States. According to Albrecht, the Rehabilitation Act of 1973 is the cornerstone of government sponsored programs for the disabled; he summarizes it as follows:

> The act: (1) established the Rehabilitation Services Administration within the Department of Health and Human Services; (2) emphasized priority treatment of those most in need, those most severely handicapped; (3) insisted that each client accepted for services be given an individualized written rehabilitation program (IWRP) to insure joint client-counselor consultation; (4) stressed consolidation and coordination of services; (5) constituted an Architectural and Transportation Barriers Compliance Board to eliminate access barriers in public places; (6) provided for affirmative action in employing the handicapped; (7) funded a national center for the deaf-blind; and increased research funding on rehabilitation. The 1978 amendments to this legislation founded the National Institute of Handicapped Research, authorized support of "independent living" facilities and programs, and offered employer incentives to train and hire the handicapped. A major theme of these legislative endeavors was to avoid institutionalization through "mainstreaming" the disabled in public life, even at considerable social and economic costs. (p. 107–108)

In the succeeding years, government funded programs have now been joined by the private sector. Albrecht argues that the "combination of large numbers of persons with disabilities, the chronicity of their conditions, and the infusion of vast sums of health insurance money to pay for rehabilitation [has led to the creation of] a gigantic new health care market in the United States" (1992, p. 134). Such a development makes it necessary for us to consider rehabilitation as a "social relationship based on the utilitarian motives of big business [as well as one based on traditional] humanitarian values" (p. 134). Both humanitarian and for-profit motives have transformed the disability business into a rehabilitation industry which has produced a division of labor and specialization in the marketplace. Albrecht says it is important "to distinguish between the fiction" that rehabilitation is an activity based on idealistic motives aimed at returning persons with disabilities to the highest possible level of functioning without regard to economic motives and the fact that "it has developed into one of the nation's most dynamic and potentially profitable industries" (1992, p. 134–135). In the previous chapter I examined the social implications of this pattern of organizing human service delivery.

Individuals with a history of employment are usually served by private, for-profit organizations. Particularly enhanced by individual and employer provided insurance programs, the private sector has grown dramatically in the past thirty years. Workers for public services have come to question the consequences for the clients who choose privately funded rehabilitation. Divergent interests have begun to contend within the rehabilitation industry. Public, not-for-profit organizations dominated service provision in the decade of the 1960s because federal resources were plentiful under Kennedy and Johnson. However, under Nixon private enterprise was encouraged and federal support was correspondingly reduced, which led to a flourishing of for-profit rehabilitation programs (Lewin, Ramseur and Fink, 1979). During the 1970s large corporations became directly involved in providing rehabilitation services for their employees (Ashton, 1979) and subsequently introduced new concerns into the rehabilitation process. State vocational agencies were interested in job placement, which sometimes required lengthy periods of formal training. According to Diamond and Petkas, "The employer/insurance carrier is seeking early closure either through job placement, which some might question as being compatible with the client's abilities and interests, or a monetary settlement" (p. 30). There was concern that the growth of private organizations in the for-profit sector would fragment the power base of the profession and confuse the public about the goals of rehabilitation. "The needs of business, industry, and government could take precedence over the needs of individual clients" (Organist, 1979, p. 54).

Despite these disagreements, rehabilitation and programs for independent living and employment, including homemaking, have a broad base of support. Autonomy, control of one's own destiny, is the goal of those experiencing rehabilitation. If a person can avoid dependency and even become self-supporting, then another tax payer is enrolled and health care costs are reduced. Professional and business leaders are pleased because old markets are expanded and new ones are opened. "The point is that rehabilitation is defined so that the interests of the state and those with power are served in meeting the needs of those with disabilities. . . . Indeed, rehabilitation, like structural responses to other social problems, evolves within and reflects the political economy and cultural values of the state" (Albrecht, 1992, p. 95).

Vocational rehabilitation, regardless of how it was to be accomplished, was the most often stated goal when political support was sought. Similarly, Albrecht describes in great detail the rapid expansion of state costs for entitlement programs related to disability and rehabilitation. "In 1986 benefits through the Social Security Disability Insurance Program to workers judged 'unable to engage in substantial gainful activity' cost 20.1 billion dollars and were supplemented by 8.8 billion dollars in medicare payments for Social Security Disability Insurance beneficiaries" (p. 104). Albrecht concludes that when all estimated costs are combined, the nation spent 169.4 billion dollars on disability related costs. In fact, the number of individuals receiving disability benefits nearly doubled from 1970 to 1980 (Matras, 1990, p. 270).

The economic costs of rehabilitation reflect inflation, continuing proliferation of professional specialization and a growing number of people seeking or requiring disability services. Approximately 9 percent of the work force in the United States, 14.2 million people, have some form of disability. Of this group, 6.3 million are limited in how much and what type of work they can do. "Some 5 percent (7.9 million) have severe work limitations, defined by the United States Bureau of the Census as not working at all or receiving Medicare or Supplemental Security Income" (United States Department of Education, 1992b). Excluding the labor force and people in institutions, approximately an additional 9.5 million Americans experience difficulty in performing daily activities (United States Department of Education, 1992a). These may be the very young or very old. Rehabilitation services to promote independent living are now included in federal funding and in the programs offered by many private agencies. Each group either requiring or receiving special assistance relates to its own group of agencies and service providers. Lane, for example, estimates that in the United States about two billion dollars is spent annually on products and services for deaf children and adults—items including special education, audiology, hearing aids, captioning devices, teletypewriters, rehabilitation and interpreter services, speech therapy and more (1992, p. 48).

Kiesler describes the economic consequences of the increasing domination of mental health programs by the medical industry. There has been a decline in community mental health outpatient programs. Mental illness is now a rapidly increasing category of disability payments. Kiesler summarizes recent changes:

...a dramatic increase in care within private psychiatric hospitals, dispro-portionately owned by hospital chains; an even more dramatic increase of psychiatric care in residential treatment centers (RTCs) for children; and a new level of organized care in general hospitals. (1992, p. 1079)

Later in this chapter I discuss the rehabilitation system as it relates to blindness.

The public sector focuses its resources on rehabilitation clients who are seeking employment for the first time and whose employability is problematic. The private sector deals with insurance claims, a large portion of work related injuries, and rehabilitation services which are supported by contractual relationships with government agencies. Additional revenues, large but difficult to determine, flow into the industry from a wide variety of professional fund raising organizations such as the United Way and associations providing money for research, support groups and rehabilitation programs for conditions such as blindness, mental illness, childhood diseases, multiple sclerosis, muscular dystrophy, and so forth. Regardless of revenue sources or auspices, rehabilitation efforts take place under a business or industrial model. From this point of view, clients are commodities to be managed and processed. The consequence of delivering rehabilitation services according to this model is the subject of the last half of this chapter.

Programs to Protect and Assist
Clients of the Rehabilitation Industry

The federal government has recognized that a unity of interest between clients of rehabilitation services and agents of these services might not always exist. In the 1970s it established a client advocacy program which, in most states, is organized as a not-for-profit corporation and which operates independently from vocational rehabilitation programs of state offices. Its purposes include assisting clients and client applicants in relationships with projects, programs, and facilities offering services. The services apply to publicly funded rehabilitation services even if contracted to private agencies. The advocacy program assists clients and client applicants in pursuing legal, administrative, and other available remedies when disputes occur (K. Kolaga, personal communication, May 7, 1992). In addition it may also advise state and other agencies of identified problem areas in the delivery of rehabilitation services.

The first protective service laws for the developmentally disabled were passed by Congress in 1975. Client assistance programs were added in 1984 as amendments to the Rehabilitation Act. Protection and advocacy services for people with mental illness were added to the program in 1987. The three programs mentioned above are based on separate statutes. Sometimes they are integrated into one program. However, in several states they operate separately under different branches of government. One branch of government has created a quasi-independent agency to assist clients as they encounter problems with government funded rehabilitation services. Protection and advocacy services themselves have become a small, but not too small, part of the rehabilitation industry. The fiscal year 1992 national budget was 9,141,000 dollars for this client protection program (B. Mitchell, personal communication, May 11, 1992).

Balancing Humanitarian and Business Interests

Organizations cannot effectively compete for scarce resources if they cannot show retained earnings or a profit.

> At the same time, no rehabilitation organization can engage in pure profit maximizing behavior without considering the social good and humanitarian values in society. Good business requires that both sets of values be considered. Therefore, both the economics of the rehabilitation marketplace and the perceived well-being of persons with disabilities have considerable effect on the organization and availability of goods and services. (Albrecht, pp. 135–136)

Regardless of the relative balance between charitable and business concerns, managers and workers are rewarded for their productivity. Accountability is an administrative concern whether the rehabilitation activity is supported by government funds, charitable organizations, or large corporations.

Components of the Industry

An organization in the rehabilitation business may be a small partnership or large corporation. It may be for-profit or not-for-profit, or a mixture of both. Sometimes it stands alone and at other times it is vertically or horizontally integrated. "Vertical integration usually refers to expansion of goods and services to encompass care that often precedes or follows hospitalization" (Albrecht, p. 136). When a group of companies producing similar products appears, an industry has been created. This condition has social consequences because the many economic interests that comprise the industry frequently merge their influence to acquire resources and control their markets. As we shall see in later chapters, these combined interest groups create ideologies and social control arrangements to manage consumers.

Albrecht makes a convincing argument for considering rehabilitation a growing industry. First, it is no longer made up of charity based organizations operating on the fringe of medical-religious organizations. Second, it is reimbursement driven. Understanding the political economy of the industry helps explain its organizational growth and diversity. If insurance will pay, services will be provided. When the government provided more money through vocational rehabilitation, Medicare, and Medicaid all kinds of providers entered the competition. Private organizations and companies compete for United Way funding. Cash flow and domain control are powerful variables in evaluating rehabilitation services. Third, a global market is developing through the standardization of products and processes, and through the use of consulting firms closely associated with funding sources and business related interest groups. For example, the People's Republic of China launched its first five-year plan for rehabilitation in 1988. The five-year plan encourages government agencies to import relevant technology and ideas from the West (Vaughan, 1992a). Fourth, as the business has grown, pressure has mounted for accountability in the public sector and for efficiency in the private sector. Finally, cooperation among administrators, professionals and even clients is necessary to demonstrate accountability and efficiency; good business requires it. Consumer groups are urged to cooperate by minimizing differences and forming coalitions to maximize support for their interests.

With the "de-industrialization" of the United States (Walton, 1990) the service sector has experienced the most rapid growth; nearly seven workers in ten are now in the service sector. Increased discretionary income, insurance programs, corporate employee benefits, annuity and pension programs, and government entitlement programs have provided money for growth in service sector employment. "The costs of just one program, Social Security benefits for the disabled, has skyrocketed from 3.1 billion in 1970 to 15.4 billion in 1980 and 20.5 billion in 1987" (Albrecht, p. 138). By 1985, approximately one dollar of every twelve public dollars spent in the United States supported programs for persons with disabilities. The number of disabled workers receiving benefits rose from 1,492,900 in 1970 to 2,858,700 in 1980 (Matras, 1990, p. 270–271). More than 80 million Americans are protected by some type of disability insurance, whether private or public. In 1968 between 120 and 160 billion dollars was paid by business and government to recipients of disability benefits (Albrecht, p. 138). The nearly doubling of the number of former workers receiving disability benefits between 1970 and 1980, as noted above, probably reflects one additional means of reducing unemployment rates or at least reducing competition for positions in the labor force. The growing number of former employees receiving disability insurance reveals a major contradiction between economic conditions and cultural values. Work is ennobling and every disabled person should have an opportunity to participate in the status and wealth conferring sector of our society. While laws prohibit discrimination, employers in the private sector have little incentive to hire the disabled if they think they will incur additional costs. Programs which once provided economic incentives to employers have been reduced, casualties of the budget cuts for human services during the past twelve years.

Of the 160 billion dollars mentioned above, significant amounts are often spent on costly, high tech rehabilitation equipment. For example, many projects have been funded by the Veterans Administration in efforts to develop technological alternatives for the sensory impaired (Koestler, 1976). Few of the expensive and complex engineering efforts described by Koestler resulted in a product that was ever widely used. Small and large companies compete to invent and market new products to enhance communication between the disabled person and his or her environment. Most are pushing computerized equipment to enhance communication and mobility. Companies continually develop new products: modified handicapped accessible vans and buses, motorized wheel chairs with multiple electronic control systems, computers with speech synthesizers connected to printers or braille printers, special electronic communication devices for the hearing impaired and prostheses of all types. Consulting companies offer advice on environmental adaptations which allegedly promote safety or accessibility. Vendors compete with the same vigor as pharmaceutical companies introducing new drugs to the market, as do professionals, advertisers, manufacturers, sales people and consumers. The passage of the Americans with Disabilities Act promises new economic opportunities for architects, interior designers, bus and van manufacturers, conference planners and conveners, lawyers, contractors, and many others.

Stakeholders

According to Albrecht, there are three major structural interests represented in this growing rehabilitation marketplace: the corporations whose business is rehabilitation, the professionals who attempt to hold monopolistic control over the delivery of rehabilitation services, and the individual and organized consumers who advocate equal access to care and quality service at a reasonable price. Government exercises control through laws and regulations directed at maintaining order in the market, serving the established structural interests, and consolidating its own power (pp. 143–144).

Some of the major players in the rehabilitation industry, those either with investment, professional or market interests, include hospitals, home health care businesses, nursing homes providing various levels of care, sheltered workshops, pharmaceutical companies, rehabilitation equipment suppliers, lawyers handling claims, appeals, and contracts, physicians who legitimate entry into the rehabilitation system, a wide array of professionals providing rehabilitation services, consulting companies, insurance companies, banks and related financial institutions which finance construction and provide other services to rehabilitation enterprises, architectural firms which design for accessibility as required by the Americans with Disabilities Act, charitable organizations which earn money from their efforts and give some of it to selected agencies, science and engineering firms developing new procedures and new products, universities receiving federal and state monies to train professionals and to provide continuing education through a constant flow of regional, state and national conferences, specialized schools for blind and deaf people and the multiply handicapped for whom "mainstreaming" is not judged appropriate, residential rehabilitation centers for diagnostic and rehabilitation activities, private agencies in most major cities providing leisure, social, educational, and sometimes employment opportunities, large national organizations representing and raising funds for all types of disabling or chronic diseases and the bureaus or divisions of every state government and territory providing vocational rehabilitation services, either directly or through private vendors, the television industry and many associated businesses which benefit directly and indirectly from telethons and other fund raising programs intended to benefit the disabled. This list could be expanded. In addition, almost every interest group on this list has its own national and regional organizations with their own professional staffs to provide continual updates about developments in the industry and to lobby for legislation relevant to particular market segments. Newsletters, journals and books about new developments appear continually.

Many consumers of rehabilitation services and other concerned citizens continually question the small amount of the wealth of this industry which actually benefits, directly or indirectly, the intended recipients. For example, the Jerry Lewis Telethon and the National Muscular Dystrophy Association, both examples of stakeholders appearing in the preceding list, are frequently the targets of criticism. Those associated with this part of the industry reap substantial economic rewards. The relatively small proportion of the proceeds which are actually applied to the stated goals has been documented (Bolte, 1992; Hershey, 1992). Almost all of the stakeholders, as I show later in this chapter, develop self-serving images of intended beneficiaries that consumers frequently judge to be harmful. Commenting on the 1992 Jerry Lewis Telethon, Bolte observes, "The negative stereotypes it creates costs America much more in bias-driven unemployment than in the piddling amounts that reaches researchers or services to the disabled. It keeps the disabled poor, segregated, and dependent" (p. 22).

As we explained in greater detail in the preceding chapter, the industrial model dominates the world of rehabilitation whether the interest is for-profit or not-for-profit. Management for economic efficiency dominates the workplace and the rehabilitation process.

> According to this model, ability to pay and projected profit margins are likely to determine who is eligible for services, the level of need, the location of treatment, the nature and intensity of the intervention programs, and new program development. Institutional managers will be influenced by selling products, marketing new programs, and turning profits in enterprises that may or may not best service those with disabilities. A growing tension exists, then, between the for-profit pressures of rehabilitation institutions and the needs of consumers with disabilities. In some instances, these forces meet and in others they are in conflict. (Albrecht, p. 178)

Industry Performance—Planned or Free Market?

The effectiveness, both in public cost and rehabilitation success for the individual, has been questioned by persons with disabilities and by other concerned citizens, including government officials (Scott, 1969; Walhof, 1984; Weaver, 1991). According to Weaver, the number of disabled people "successfully rehabilitated," capable of being suitably employed, has declined by 25 percent in the last twelve years.

In her 1992 address to the national convention of the National Federation of the Blind, Nell Carney, Commissioner of the Rehabilitation Services Administration, commented on the failure of rehabilitation services to result in competitive employment. "I did look at the statistics last year for blind and visually impaired people served by public vocational rehabilitation and found that only 35 percent of the cases closed were closed in competitive employment. That figure is absolutely unacceptable to us at the Rehabilitation Services Administration" (p. 593). She also indicated that, in the future, evaluation of the efficacy of federally funded rehabilitation programs should focus on outcomes rather than process. She also favored additional choice in regard to the selection of rehabilitation providers. In a 1991 report to Congress based on 1988 data gathered by the Rehabilitation Services Administration, significant questions were raised about the long term effectiveness of rehabilitation programs. The study showed that for clients re-employed after rehabilitation services, earnings soon dropped below pre-vocational rehabilitation levels. "The average earnings for those working did go up each year; however, eight years after rehabilitation, forty percent still had annual earnings that totaled less than the equivalent of working all year at the minimum wage" (York, 1991, p. 2). The report reflects earnings based on the week before referral and earnings after rehabilitation—that is, after renewed employment for sixty days. All the data is based on rigorous data obtained by the General Accounting Office and includes Social Security earnings for the three years before vocational rehabilitation services were received. The study monitored 266,176 clients and their earning histories from the same data sources which were analyzed for eight years following their re-employment for these same individuals (pp. 2–6).

Weaver claims the weakness of the rehabilitation program is the absence of competition. Federal and state funded programs and their contractual partners dominate the rehabilitation process. Not only does minimal competition enable more established programs to grab funds, but there is little freedom of choice for the individual requiring rehabilitation services.

Physicians determine eligibility and state agencies or privately employed professionals diagnose the potential for rehabilitation, provide direct services, and contract with private providers for additional services. In a great many cases, social networks develop between public providers and private contractors, which increases the likelihood of similar program philosophies being linked economically. Although the private sector may be involved, it is not a free market. A client requiring public assistance, in most cases, may not go to a program of choice but to one currently under contract with a state agency. Some have argued that a voucher system be used for vocational rehabilitation such as the one being considered for public education. "Vocational rehabilitation agencies would be responsible for making basic eligibility decisions, but beyond that, they would have to compete on a fee-for-service basis. Diversity in rehabilitation approaches would be encouraged in a system built on decentralized decision-making, competition, and choice" (Weaver, p. 22). As we will see in greater detail later in this book, Weaver anticipates resistance to a "free market" approach. Rehabilitation counselors may resist because their employment security has been related to publicly funded and managed programs. Opposition will also come from large private agencies that have come to depend on a steady flow of revenue under present arrangements. According to Weaver, state administrators of rehabilitation programs, and there are many within each state, control large resources and many employment and career opportunities.

> Surely they will argue that public vocational rehabilitation counselors are the only ones with the qualifications necessary to make complex and important decisions regarding service regimen and supplies. And surely it will be implied, if not stated outright, that those in need of vocational rehabilitation services are poorly suited to protect their own interests. (pp. 22–23)

A voucher system, or some other means providing alternatives for consumers, would enable individuals seeking rehabilitation services to avoid the agencies or programs they judge to be harmful or less effective. Competition might produce more alternatives. As in the medical industry in general, competition might actually increase, rather than reduce, costs. However, to restate an earlier observation, the dependency creating aspects of rehabilitation programs occur regardless of the source of funding. As we saw in the preceding chapter, dependency is a consequence of dealing with bureaucratic organizations which operate according to the norms of rational efficiency.

The Blindness Rehabilitation Business

All that has been said about the disability industry applies equally well to the field of blindness rehabilitation, which is a subset of the general enterprise. As we will see later in greater detail, its advocates argue that blindness is such a severe disability that it requires its own specialized professionals and agencies. It receives designated funding from both federal and state governments, and there are more than five hundred private agencies in the United States which specialize in dealing with people with visual handicaps. Workers for the blind have their own journals, annual national and international meetings, university training centers, vendors of adaptive technology, and professional organizations. Most organizations of blind people support this separateness as being necessary.

In most states the business of rehabilitating blind people is organizationally and programmatically separate from the general vocational rehabilitation program. Despite the intentional separation, this sector of the industry demonstrates the same economic linkages among public funding sources, private businesses, and not-for-profit corporations.

Determining the economic cost of rehabilitation programs for blind people is difficult because funding comes from many different sources. People who are blind may have other problems unrelated to blindness that require rehabilitation and may receive services from more than one agency or program. A 1967 national survey reported that federal funds accounted for 57 percent of expenditures, the private sector 15 percent, and state programs 28 percent (Organization for Social and Technical Innovation, Inc., 1971). Unfortunately, this study was unable to identify federal funds which may have flowed through private agencies. A 1982 national survey of services for the blind and visually impaired reported that 195 relatively large agencies had a combined budget of 222.4 million dollars (Kirchner, 1983a). However, the survey did not include the budgets of more than four hundred additional agencies.

Although the data is more than twenty years old, a report prepared for the U.S. Department of Health, Education, and Welfare in 1976 illustrates the costs and the variety of groups who benefited from dealing with persons affected by sensory loss. The report also includes several reasons why these numbers were conservative estimates, and I have found no plausible way to determine what they might be today because of the inflation rate of health costs in the United States, the aging of the labor force with increased incidents of sensory decline, the proliferation of medical and rehabilitation professionals providing services, and the greater variety of rehabilitation programs. The following chart from the 1976 report reflects the disbursement of revenue in the medical-rehabilitation industry related to blindness (Cahill, 1976, p. 6).

Manufacturing the Product

The business of rehabilitation is conducted in diverse settings. Rehabilitation for a blind person may begin, after eligibility has been determined, with an evaluation in a residential evaluation center. The

Summary of Estimates of the Economic Costs of
Visual Disorders and Disabilities: United States, 1972

Category of Expenditures or loss	Expenditures or Losses (in millions of dollars)
Direct Costs	
Visits to Ophthalmologists	$ 352.5
Visits to Other M.D.'s	50.1
Eye Surgery	273.7
Optometrists' Services and Materials	1,196.7
In-patient Hospital Care	336.8
Nursing Home Care	829.3
Ophthalmic Drugs and Optical Goods	564.6
Total	$3,603.7
Indirect Costs (Loss of Earnings)	
Days Lost from Work (acute episodes)	$ 105.4
Persons Unable to Work	775.9
Women Unable to Keep House	184.7
Institutionalized Persons	419.2
Total	$1,485.2

center may operate under contract from a state rehabilitation agency, with a large number of clients "going through the process" at any given time. Different kinds of professional workers evaluate each client's intelligence, level of social adjustment, ability to travel, general appearance and grooming skills, personality, and vocational interests as the client understands them at that point in time.

The facilities may be quite large and well funded as, for example, are the rehabilitation centers supported by the Veterans Administration. According to Albrecht, "V.A. rehabilitation programs are situated in huge government bureaucracies where services are viewed as due every disabled veteran who served with honor. The cost or functional accountability is slight and no rush exists to move patients through the system and back to home and job. The system is largely paternalistic in culture" (Albrecht, p. 264). When I asked one recipient of Veterans Administration rehabilitation services for blindness to share his impressions of the V.A. centers, he laughingly said, "You need to bring a van or truck with you to carry home all of the gadgets you will receive." Another respondent described this setting as having plenty of money and technology — everything but a positive philosophy about blindness.

From the wealth of resources of the V.A. system, the other extreme is a solo itinerant practitioner visiting a client's home to teach braille, cane travel or independent living skills. Such visits occur only in the context of formally established procedures including mutually agreed upon goals between client, contract provider, and the state agency paying for the services.

Regardless of the size and bureaucratic complexity of any rehabilitation setting, the stakeholders participate in a similar procedure: a professional worker determines eligibility, evaluates the client, and initiates a program intended to lead to employment or, in some cases, independent living. This seems to be an efficient, expedient, and benevolent method for treating the blind.

> Although most often cast as purchasers of services, consumers are also raw material and finished products in the rehabilitation industry. In the rehabilitation system, consumers are the raw material to which value is added for a price. By definition, an individual with a disability has lost function. Rehabilitation experts strive to assist the individual to recapture that lost function through participation in a treatment regimen. The outcome of successful intervention is improved performance signifying a person more valued in society. (Albrecht, p. 298)

Throughout the resulting procedures, the person is a case to be processed by the various workers involved. The client may spend many hours doing nothing while awaiting events scheduled for the convenience of the organization. The person seeking rehabilitation may be anxious, uncertain as to how he or she is being perceived and aware that the process is "the only game in town." Quite normal and ordinary procedures from the point of view of the organization may appear to the client as silly, unnecessary, demeaning and seemingly endless. The client feels himself or herself continually being considered as a type or category of a problem rather than as a whole person. The notion of "red tape" is used universally to describe the frustration ordinary citizens feel in dealing with bureaucratic requirements, and there is a full measure of it here.

In a setting where uncertainty and anxiety are frequently present and where the client feels powerless and has to "play the game," organizational procedures can be particularly distressing. The personal conceptions a client brings to the rehabilitation setting may have little to do with what follows. As Scott noted, counselors often define blindness as a severe problem requiring intensive, long-term intervention. Much energy is devoted to changing the client's view of what he or she "needs." "Discrediting the client's personal ideas about his problem is achieved in several ways. His initial statements about why he has come to the organization and what he hopes to receive from it are euphemistically termed 'the presenting problem,' a phrase that implies superficiality in the client's view" (1969, p. 77). Subsequent testing, observation, and counseling may lead to recommendations for long term involvement in the prescribed programs. Questioning these may in turn raise questions of "maladjustment" and "denial." As Albrecht (1992) notes, economic concerns resulting in a production process influences the outcome which follows the intake interview. The rehabilitation business, at this point, can affect the client's future. Organizational concerns rooted in economic imperatives influence policies and programs that continually require raw material for processing.

In dealing with organizational procedures, blind people do not have the luxury of being "ordinary" as other people are ordinary. As noted above, there is a limited market for pursuing alternatives. The client quickly learns that making a pleasing impression on these various examiners is extremely important. To question the process or, by any means, to question the superordinate position of a staff member will not advance one's interests. To many, the loss of social and psychological independence is not worth the cost (Zola, 1983).

As a former client, I have experienced this process myself. As a sociologist, on one recent occasion I spent two weeks in an evaluation center observing the procedures as clients were evaluated. My experience included residing with the clients in the residential center. I observed the "underlife" of blind people experiencing rehabilitation (Goffman, 1961). Students or clients make jokes or laugh at the "counselors." They also share strategies for manipulating or dealing with the process. However, as individuals, they seldom question their subordinate position in the relationship. One example of what occurs when one challenges a counselor is illustrated by a client whose condition was other than blindness. Lucy Gwin, as reported by Albrecht, describes a scenario similar to those in which many other handicapped people have participated.

> Therapist Ann Patrice approached me at the picnic table behind the day facility one morning. "We have to do something about getting you some bras," she said. "I don't wear bras," I told her. "Well, you need some bras, and there's no money in your account. Wouldn't it be fun to go shopping for some bras?" I told her I'd like to go shopping for a toothbrush, toothpaste, shampoo, nail file, SOAP! That I hadn't worn bras since I was 15 when brassieres were a status

symbol. That bras are uncomfortable, that my breasts are small enough to survive without "support." "We'll have to ask your daughter to send money for your personal account so you can get some bras." I told her that if the money materialized, and bras were forced on me, I would cut them into small pieces. She asked me if I was making a threat of some kind, a threat of bodily harm to her. No, I told her, it's you who are threatening to put my tits in prison.

Shortly after this encounter, Lucy Gwin's records showed that she had threatened the therapist; that she was a "difficult" patient. Such patients judged to be obstinate are frequently deprived of privileges and sometimes even refused therapy. (p. 265)

Similar incidents are frequently reported in the consumer literature. For example, Paul Burkhardt described his response to his rehabilitation counselor's interest in the tidiness of his apartment. The counselor also chided the client for using his own initiative in seeking employment. "In that same conversation Mr. Hackinson pulled no punches when he told me not to contact Wang Laboratories on my own for employment inquiries, but to leave that to the Commission" (1984, p. 428). After reviewing Mr. Burkhardt's letter of complaint, the director of the Massachusetts Commission for the Blind responded as follows: "The representations made by your counselor in reference to the tidiness of your home were made in conjunction with enhancement of your organizational skills" (Crawford, 1984, p. 555). The commissioner went on to interpret the client's complaints as a "misperception of our attitude" (p. 556). The concept of custodialism as illustrated by this incident is developed further at the end of this chapter.

While an undergraduate student at West Virginia University in 1957, I was receiving vocational rehabilitation assistance for part of my college expenses. This included thirty-two dollars per semester towards the cost of textbooks. Enrolled in a course on philosophies of India, I was required to purchase a text entitled *A White Umbrella.* After the bookstore billed the appropriate vocational rehabilitation office, a formal letter was sent to university officials indicating that if Mr. Vaughan needed a white umbrella, he would have to buy it himself. No one bothered to ask me about the item they were questioning. It was much ado about nothing and, at the time, seemed humorous to me. However, in the intervening thirty-six years, I have more than once recalled this incident. If rehabilitation is indeed a partnership, in this instance not only was I ignored, my integrity was questioned and another bureaucracy, the university, was needlessly involved. Had I made an issue of this event, I would almost certainly have been told that I was too sensitive or did not adequately appreciate concerns for fiscal accountability.

Zygmut Bauman (1988) summarizes the situation of the heteronomous individual who confronts power in the context of the formally organized human service delivery system.

> The bureaucratic determination of needs means a persistent lack of personal autonomy and individual freedom. Heteronomy of life is what constitutes deprivation in a consumer society. The life of the deprived is subject to bureaucratic regimentation, which isolates and incapacitates its victims, leaving them little chance to fight back, answer back, or even resist through noncooperation. In the life of the deprived, politics is omnipresent and omnipotent; it penetrates deeply into the most private areas of one's existence, while at the same time remaining distant, alien and inaccessible. The bureaucrats "see without being seen"; they speak and expect to be heard, but hear only what they think is worth hearing; they reserve the right to draw the line between the true need and a mere whim, between prudence and prodigality, reason and unreason, the "normal" and the "insane." (p. 85–86)

Deference and compliance are presumed—the natural due to those of superior knowledge and training (Larson, 1977, p. 157).

The Consumer as Part of the Industry

As I have already mentioned, the number of alternatives available to people seeking rehabilitation services is usually limited. Being a customer, or consumer, implies a relationship with the organization or business providing the service. Customers are technically on the outside. "The organization has no authority over its customers although it may try to tie them to the organization in several ways, through special price reductions and other favors" (Ahrne, 1991, p. 40).

The relationship of customer and business, to continue this metaphor, defies neat, organizational classification. The consumer of rehabilitation services is influenced more by the business or agency than is the customer buying shoes or compact discs. Not only is the consumer limited in choice, the involvement is frequently intensive. The consumer may experience a prolonged period of involvement with a service delivery agency before attaining a glimpse of the outcome (Swaan, 1990). He or she can not easily put the involvement back on the shelf. The customer has frequently entered an heteronomous situation. In principle, the consumer is an autonomous agent. In fact, the greater the involvement with agencies of rehabilitation, the greater the likelihood of becoming a product—being molded and managed to fit the agency's procedures and processes (Scott, 1969). Agencies delight in finding attractive consumers—those who are compliant and can be presented as successful products as agencies compete for scarce resources. Youth, a pleasing appearance, the proper demeanor, and good prospects for future community involvement and employment are among the most desirable characteristics. When such consumers respond positively to organizational management, social recognition and other small benefits, occasionally even a job, come their way.

Scott (1969) describes the importance of attractive clients for agency-community relationships. Those who contribute money, as Scott notes, usually know little about blindness and have no perspective for judging the consequences of agency activity. To maximize resource acquisition,

> Clients are carefully selected, the encounters are short, and the social roles played by participants are highly stereotyped. A distinctive emotional climate pervades these meetings, consisting of a subtle blend of pathos, amiability, gratitude, wonder, praise, humor, and tension. Typically, blind clients make a statement concerning their plight before coming to an agency for help, the kinds of help they have received, the changes the agency has brought about in their lives, the happiness that is now there, and the gratitude they feel toward the agency and its benefactors. Such testimonials comprise a major part of the contact that occurs between blind clients and the community (pp. 91–92).

Our communities support businesses and public agencies that "take care of" blind people, many of whom fall into a pattern of becoming dependent upon agencies for leisure, social activities, and even employment opportunities. There is even greater economic gain for the agency if an employed worker can produce well in the sheltered shop at substandard wages; more funds will be available for other purposes. The consumer hopes for, and agency rhetoric speaks of, independence, self-reliance, competing on an equal basis for employment opportunity, and full participation in society. As this book will demonstrate, the opposite is often the outcome. As Scott observed, "In fact, the blind person who deliberately thrusts himself into the everyday life of the community is soon treated as a nuisance, and the blindness worker who pursues too seriously the avowed goal of reintegration soon wears out his welcome in the community" (p. 92).

With the specialization of social control agencies many ordinary citizens come to expect agencies to be "the place" to take care of blind people. For example, Aubrey Webson (1992) describes a situation in which a blind, young radio disc jockey was found intoxicated by the police. The police took the man not to his apartment or to jail, but to the agency that serves blind people. More importantly, Webson observes that they did not treat him as they would have treated ordinary drunks because they did not know how to deal with him. This lack of experience with independent, self-reliant blind people underlies the consistently high level of political support for public programs for blind people and the seeming ease with which charitable contributions can be extracted from the concerned public.

The Organized Blind

As Albrecht notes, succeeding cohorts of consumers have become increasingly reflective about their common situation.

> These better informed consumers are shaping the market through the exercise of their knowledge, purchasing power, and insistence on being included in decision making. In the disability arena, growing numbers of clients are demanding rehabilitation and public accessibility as rights. They realize that they do not have to be hidden in custodial institutions or their parents' homes (pp. 278–279).

Consumer consciousness developed around different disability groups. Organized groups began social movements which challenged the knowledge base of professionals and questioned the adequacy or benevolence of service delivery systems. According to Haug and Sussman (1969), the 1960s was the decade of the consumer revolt, whether in education, poverty programs, or other human service delivery programs. Rather than dropping out, citizens began to organize and demand equal participation. The authors list four situations in which scrutiny of professional autonomy is justified:

> 1) the expertise of the practitioners is inadequate, 2) their claims to altruism are unfounded, 3) the organizational delivery system supporting their authority is defective and insufficient or 4) this system is too efficient and exceeds the appropriate bounds of its power. (p. 156)

For these reasons and others mentioned below, organizations of blind people challenged those in charge of their sector of the disability industry. However, in the United States, this challenge predated the 1960s by at least 20 years. The occupational group, Work for the Blind, was challenged before it even began to call itself a profession. As we will see in Chapters 5 and 6 as professionals sought greater control, consumer resistance intensified.

Organizations of blind people, namely guilds, have been described in many parts of the world for more than one thousand years (Vaughan and Vaughan, 1993). Approximately two hundred years ago, and more recently in the United States, special institutions were created to provide custodial care and education for blind people. Preparing people for employment was thought to be good for the blind person and useful for society. However, these institutions were economically insignificant for the wider society, and the occupational status of caretakers and superintendents was low.

Gradually, in this century public support, legislation, and funding began to make possible more education and, finally, vocational rehabilitation training for blind people. This progress always included goals such as full participation in society, economic security, equal treatment, and autonomy. It is not surprising that many, very ordinary, blind people took these goals to heart. Why not? Are these not goals equally lauded for all citizens? Thoughtful blind people became concerned when they saw their opportunities being diminished by what they took to be paternalistic, custodial, and dependency creating aspects of their experiences with educational and rehabilitation services.

Ironically, the very schools and agencies themselves brought blind people together. The factory was an invention of the industrial revolution and this new physical work place brought laborers together in common work settings and nearby housing. Each worker readily saw that his or her plight was not unique. Leaders emerged to develop unions for improved conditions. Perhaps I have stretched the analogy too far; however, the forerunners of the present rehabilitation industry brought blind people together, and began to assist them in their education and to affirm goals to which no one could object.

In 1940 the first national organization of blind people was established— the National Federation of the Blind. During the previous two decades, federal monies were being appropriated, agency specializations were developing among those who worked for the blind, and agencies were proliferating. From the earliest days of organizations of blind people in this country, concerns for employment opportunities and equal treatment were paramount. The first president of the Federation, Jacobus tenBroek consistently argued for blind people's right of self-determination.

> For if we cannot say that "bad men" have combined against us, we can and do say that men of bad philosophy and little faith have done so—sighted and sightless men whose vision is short, whose ears are stopped, and whose minds are closed by institutional and occupational self-interest, whose banner is the

wretched patchwork of medieval charity and poor relief. (cited in Matson, 1990, p. 74–75)

Dr. tenBroek also called for a bill of rights for blind people—that their freedom and autonomy should be the same as for any other citizen.

Jacobus tenBroek was a professor at the University of California, Berkeley and a recognized scholar in the area of civil rights and welfare reform. His books dealt with issues related to the 14th amendment, the forced relocation of Japanese Americans during World War II, family law, and issues of civil rights (tenBroek, 1951, 1955; tenBroek and Handler, 1971; tenBroek and Matson, 1968). Professor tenBroek saw clearly many of the contradictions between the interests of rehabilitation agencies and the educational needs of blind people. He observed that the blending of welfare and educational issues were frequently not in the interest of blind people. He brought a scholarly background in the area of civil rights along with his own experience as a blind citizen to his leadership of the first national organization of blind people.

This social movement of blind people grew rapidly and soon spread to every state in the United States. Its leaders and members challenged what they judged to be unjust practices and harmful attitudes about blindness. A detached observer might reasonably think that agency officials and rehabilitation workers would applaud these accomplishments and perhaps even take a little credit. With many notable exceptions, the opposite has been the case. This consumer movement encountered increasing resistance as it questioned many of the practices of the rehabilitation industry. Did the industry create the opposition movement?

Blind people are socialized—they learn to respond according to how other people think about them and act toward them. The social nature of blindness is defined by the expectations of others, not by the amount of sensory loss experienced by each individual. Certainly, participation in the rehabilitation service delivery system has caused some blind people to think of themselves and their situations in political terms. They have common problems, consciousness of which in a democracy reasonably leads to political action. The separate service systems created for blind people have helped bring into focus their common grievances.

Social movements focus on grievances; the worst aspects of the blindness industry were denounced and picketed. Focusing on conflicts can help clarify patterns of domination. Holders of political and economic resources, including cultural transmission institutions, are the focus of our efforts to understand persistently enduring structures of relationships which alter the life chances of subordinate groups (Adam, 1978, p. 4). The National Federation of the Blind acquired notoriety as it confronted traditional practices and those who directed agencies and programs. Its demand that blind people should speak for themselves contradicted ideas that many professionals and educators held concerning limitations caused by blindness. The principle of self-determination was not negotiable. Any practice where agency or agency personnel benefited from the surplus value created by the labor of blind workers was not acceptable. Concern over exploitation of workers in sheltered workshops has continued to be a major consumer concern.

In 1971 Kenneth Jernigan, the president (following Dr. tenBroek) of the organized blind movement in the United States, sent a clear message to the agencies in which he explained the organization's philosophy concerning who should decide issues affecting blind people.

> If you tell us that you are important and necessary to our lives, we reply: It is true. But tear down every agency for the blind in the nation, destroy every workshop, and burn every professional journal; and we can build them all back if they are needed. But take away the blind, and your journals will go dusty on the shelves. Your counselors will walk the streets for work, and your broomcorn will mold and rot in your sheltered shops. Yes, we need you; but you need us too. We intend to have a voice in your operation and your decisions since what you do affects our lives. We intend to have representation on your boards, and we intend for you to recognize our organizations and treat us as equals. We are not your wards, and there is no way for you to make us your wards. The only question left to be answered is whether you will accept the new conditions and work with us in peace and partnership or whether we must drag you kicking and screaming into the new era. But enter the new era you will, like it or not. (cited in Matson, 1990, p. 749)

Critics, usually associated with major agencies and professional leaders of the rehabilitation business, frequently tried to discredit or co-opt the leadership. A continual refrain was that this consumer organization did not represent all or even most blind people. In one sense they were correct. However, neither do political parties in the United States represent all citizens. Voter turnout is low and millions are not registered as voters, yet democratic political processes are available. From its beginnings the Federation was organized on democratic principles with local, state, and national arenas for participation. Roughly, including officers of local chapters and their elected boards, state affiliates, national divisions, and so forth, there are at least five thousand elected positions in the

National Federation of the Blind (Vaughan, 1992b). It has grown despite splits and severe internal conflicts, and continues to be a strong advocate for blind people in the battle with the rehabilitation industry. I have argued, as has Albrecht (1992), that the consumer is an integral part of the rehabilitation industry, and organizations created by consumers play no less a part. In fact, they become formal organizations with economic resources. For example, the National Federation of the Blind through its membership, raised a budget in excess of eight million dollars in 1992. This figure does not include monies raised in local chapters and state affiliates which totals several million dollars more (M. Maurer, personal communication, August 21, 1992). The national headquarters, the National Center for the Blind in Baltimore, Maryland, has forty employees and occupies one city block with more than 200,000 square feet of space. The national center includes a conference center, publications distribution operation, a national technology center and an aids and appliances distribution center. The monthly journal, the *Braille Monitor,* has a circulation exceeding thirty thousand. Organizations of consumers have become major interest groups representing economic and political resources which have influenced changes in the practices of the rehabilitation business.

In the United States many blind people have made contributions to the developing concerns for autonomy and self-determination. The first person to achieve national prominence was Professor Jacobus tenBroek, the founder and first president of the National Federation of the Blind. In this book, I frequently talk about structures, organizations, interest groups—even industries. Such general concepts should not cause us to disregard the personalities and events which have influenced the developments under review. Individual agencies and the conflict as seen from the point of view of the actors are equally important. Most agree that no one was more involved in the events which this book discusses than were Dr. Jacobus tenBroek and Dr. Kenneth Jernigan, author of the following memorial to Dr. tenBroek.

JACOBUS tenBROEK—THE MAN AND THE MOVEMENT

If my remarks today were to have a title, it might well be: "Jacobus tenBroek—The Man and the Movement." For the relationship of this man to the organized blind movement, which he brought into being in the United States and around the world, was such that it would be equally accurate to say that the man was the embodiment of the movement or that the movement was the expression of the man.

For tens of thousands of blind Americans over more than a quarter of a century he was leader, mentor, spokesman, and philosopher. He gave to the organized blind movement the force of his intellect and the shape of his dreams. He made it the symbol of a cause barely imagined before his coming: the cause of self-expression, self-direction and self-sufficiency on the part of blind people. Step by step, year by year, action by action, he made that cause succeed.

There are those who will tell you it all started in Wilkes-Barre, Pennsylvania in 1940 when the blind of seven states came together to organize. But they are wrong. It started much earlier in the age-old discriminations against the blind, in the social ostracism, the second-class citizenship, and the denial of opportunity—it started in primitive times before the first recorded history, in the feelings of the community at large and the restiveness of the blind, the wish for improvement, the resistance to a system.

Its seeds were there when the first schools for the blind were founded in America in the 1800's, when the first feeble beginnings of rehabilitation occurred in the present century—in the increasing numbers of blind college students, in the ever-expanding agencies established to serve the blind, in the custodialism, the hope, the frustration, the despair, and the courage.

But it also started on July 6, 1911, on the prairies of Alberta, Canada. On that date in that place was born Jacobus tenBroek. His father was a strong-willed "renegade" Dutchman who first asserted his own independence by running away from home at seven to become a cabin boy. Over the next thirty years he literally sailed the seven seas and roamed most of the world, but at the ripe age of forty he felt a hankering to settle down. Through devious negotiations with the Dutch community in California he arranged a marriage with a girl whom he met for the first time on their wedding day—and promptly took up homesteading in the rugged Canadian prairies of Alberta. Like his fellow "sodbusters" of that era, Nicolaas tenBroek earned the right to own his section (640 acres) of hard ground through arduous years of clearing and breaking it. But unlike the other homesteaders, who customarily constructed their huts out of the native sod, Elder tenBroek chose to build his home of logs chopped from the tall Alberta timber.

In that primitive, dirt-floor cabin, both Jacobus and his older brother Nicolaas were born. Some years later when the worst edge of grinding poverty had been turned, their father set about erecting the first frame house to be seen in that part of the province. But the rustic log cabin still stands today, hardly the worse for more than a half-century of wear—as a monument to Dutch craftsmanship and North American timber.

One day, seven-year-old Jacobus and a boyhood friend were playing at bows and arrows, taking turns aiming at a roughly-constructed bull's eye cut out of a large piece of canvas. On a sudden whim, young tenBroek darted behind the cloth to peer through the hole at his companion. At that moment the other boy released an arrow from his bow—and for once that day the missile was perfectly on target.

The sight of one eye was irrevocably lost to Jacobus tenBroek on that afternoon. Even then, however, had he received prompt and expert medical attention he would have retained the full sight of the other eye. But in rural Alberta in those days, such care was not to be had. Before many years had gone by Jacobus was totally blind.

Perhaps it required the challenge of blindness to get his "Dutch" up. At any rate, the stubborn streak of independence he had inherited from both parents, coupled with a spartan upbringing on a prairie homestead prevented any lapse into helplessness or self-pity. The family decided to move back to California so that Jacobus could enroll in the California School for the Blind. Following this schooling he enrolled in the University of California, where he graduated with highest honors and went on to win the Order of the Coif at the University Law School.

In 1937 he won what he was to consider his greatest triumph: the hand of his wife, Hazel. The three children and the happy life which followed gave evidence to the wisdom of that judgement.

The question has been put before: What if that fateful arrow had never flown? But the arrow did fly and the results are a matter of history. Jacobus tenBroek went on to earn five college degrees, including a doctorate from Harvard and another from the University of California. He became a brilliant teacher and scholar, a renowned author, and a prominent authority in the field of social welfare. He also became the founder and leader of the National Federation of the Blind. From the very beginning the organization was active, tumultuous, dynamic, inspiring. It struggled, prospered, had civil war, and re-built.

And through it all, one man was a central figure—Jacobus tenBroek. His enemies called him a tyrant, and hated him. His friends called him Chick and loved him.

I first met Chick in 1952, when the Federation was twelve years old. From that time until his death he was my closest friend—my teacher, companion, counselor, colleague, and brother. I worked with him in good times and in bad, and had occasion to know him in every conceivable kind of situation. He could be harsh and quick of temper, but he could also be gentle, considerate, and generous. He was the greatest man I have ever known.

When he began the Federation in 1940 the plight of the blind was sorry, indeed. To start any organization at all was a monumental effort. It involved finding and stimulating blind people, licking stamps and cranking the mimeograph machine, finding funds and resources, and doing battle with the agencies bent on perpetuating custodialism.

When I came on the scene in 1952, the Federation was a going concern. The convention was held in New York that year, and we had our first nationwide coverage—a fifteen minute tenBroek speech. The early and mid-fifties were a time of growth and harmony for the organized blind movement. New states were joining the Federation; money was coming into the treasury; and we established our magazine, *THE BRAILLE MONITOR*. By 1956 the organization had reached full maturity. Almost a thousand delegates gathered at San Francisco to hear a classic statement of the hopes, purposes and problems of the blind. It was Dr. tenBroek's banquet address, "Within the Grace of God." His address the following year at New Orleans—"The Cross of Blindness" and "The Right of the Blind to Organize"—were equally cogent.

Shortly after the New Orleans convention, smoldering sparks of conflict within the Federation flamed into open civil war. The three succeeding conventions—Boston in 1958, Santa Fe in 1959, and Miami in 1960—left the organization in virtual ruin. What had been a great crusade had now become a bickering political movement. Unity was gone; and although the overwhelming majority of the members still believed in the leadership of Dr. tenBroek, they seemed unable to mobilize themselves to meet this new type of challenge. The opposition established a magazine, calling it the "Free Press." There were character assassinations, charges and countercharges. When Dr. tenBroek rose to speak to the delegates at the Kansas City convention in 1961, his voice was weary, and his work carried sorrow and defeat. He cited two lists of occurrences during the preceding year—things the Federation had done, and things that had been done to the Federation—by its own disruptive faction from within. He said that he had undergone extreme and bitter personal attack, aimed at destroying his career and his reputation. "They have called me a Hitler," he said, "a Stalin and a Mussolini. They have compared me to Caesar." He then told the audience that he felt that he had no choice but to resign. As he talked, the dissenters shifted uneasily in their seats, the majority wept. When he finished, I walked off of that stage with him and it seemed to me as if the organized blind movement might be finished.

But the Federation did not die. From those dark days of 1961 it rallied. The resignation of Dr. tenBroek seemed to galvanize the members into action. The dissenters were expelled. Renewal and rebirth began. The 1962 convention at Detroit was a welcome contrast to the four which had preceded it. Although Dr. tenBroek was not the president, he was still the spiritual leader of the movement. This fact was made clear by his reception throughout the meeting and, particularly, at the banquet, where he delivered the principal address.

In 1965 the Federation met in the nation's Capital. The convention was tumultuous, enthusiastic. The Vice President of the United States spoke, as did the Speaker of the House and numerous others. The climax came at the banquet when more than one hundred congressmen and senators came to the packed hotel ballroom to hear one of the truly great tenBroek speeches.

In the history of every movement there are crucial events and landmark years. 1966 was such for the Federation. When the delegates met at Louisville, there was an air of expectancy. On the afternoon of the first day, President Russell Kletzing rose to make his report. He summarized the past four years of organizational development and concluded by saying that he would not be a candidate for re-election. Then it was moved that Dr. tenBroek be elected to the presidency by acclamation. There was pandemonium. As on that other day in Kansas City, the majority wept. It was a day of complete re-dedication and renewal.

This was in July. In August Dr. tenBroek learned that he had cancer. The surgery which followed brought hope, waiting, and ultimate disappointment. As the year progressed and the pain grew, the end seemed inevitable. He came to the 1967 convention at Los Angeles in high good humor and tranquility. It was his last. There are many who say it was his greatest. When he rose to make the banquet address, it seemed a fitting climax and valedictory.

In the fall of 1967 surgery was again necessary. The cancer was widespread and incurable. On March 27, 1968, Jacobus tenBroek died. During his years he lived more and accomplished more than most men ever can or do. He was the source of love for his family, joy for his friends, consternation for his opponents and hope for the disadvantaged. He moved the blind from immobility to action, from silence to expression, from degradation to dignity—and through that movement he moved a nation.

"No greater summation of his philosophy can be given than his own concluding words in his speech "Within the Grace of God.""

"In the 16th century John Bradford made a famous remark which has ever since been held up to us as a model of Christian humility and great charity. Seeing a beggar in his rags, creeping along a wall through a flash of lightening in a stormy night, Bradford said: 'But for the Grace of God, there go I.' Compassion was shown; pity was shown; charity was shown; humility was shown; there was even an acknowledgement that the relative positions of the two could and might have been switched. Yet despite the compassion, despite the pity, despite the charity, despite the humility, how insufferably arrogant! There was still an unbridgeable gulf between Bradford and the beggar. They were not one but two. Whatever might have been, Bradford thought himself Bradford and the beggar a beggar—one high, the other low; one wise, the other misguided; one strong, the other weak; one virtuous, the other depraved.

We do not and we cannot take the Bradford approach. It is not just that beggary is the badge of our past and is still all too often the present symbol of social attitudes towards us; although that is at least part of it. But in the broader sense, we are that beggar, and he is each of us. We are made in the same image and of the same ingredients. We have the same weaknesses and strengths, the same feelings, emotions, and drives; and we are products of the same social economic, and other environmental forces. How much more a part of true humanity, to say instead: 'There, within the Grace of God, do go I.' "

So Chick spoke in a graphic pronouncement. On another occasion he said: "Movements are built of principles and of men. Movements without principles should not exist. Movements with principles—

but without men of energy, intelligence and training to give them life—cannot exist."

He was such a man. He gave to the movement all that he had—his time, his energy, and his love. The only thing he took in return was such satisfaction as he derived from his labors. In the hearts of blind men and women throughout America and the world, his memory lives, and will live. In the life and work of Jacobus tenBroek can be read the story of a man and a movement. (1968, pp. 29–34)

Throughout this book I illustrate events or conditions with lengthy quotes from the people involved. I have not neglected the leadership, but have intentionally selected material from a variety of ordinary, run of the mill blind people. They comprise the thousands of individuals who have constituted the social movement described in this book. Their efforts, plus leadership, were the force behind the early growth of the organized blind. Their efforts, plus leadership, were the force behind the early growth of the organized blind movement which has been thoroughly documented by Floyd Matson (1990).

THE DARK AGES—AND THE DAWN ORGANIZATION

Inevitably, the nationalizing of welfare led to the nationalizing of the organized blind movement. Various factors, internal and external to the movement, combined in this preliminary period to nourish a growing sense of brotherhood, of common needs and aspirations, both among blind students mingling in their residential state schools and among blind workers meeting and sharing grievances in their all-too-sheltered workshops. A powerful rallying cry emerged during the course of the Depression decade in the form of the struggle to "save Social Security from the Social Security Board"—that is, to protect blind recipients of aid from the means test and other onerous conditions newly imposed by the federal agency. The campaign to salvage and reform the program of aid to the blind, and in so doing to transform relief into rehabilitation, was to dominate the agenda of the National Federation of the Blind at its founding convention and to remain a guiding theme through its first decade. (pp. iii–v)

The following article from the *Braille Monitor* as reprinted from the *Buffalo News* illustrates several aspects of business resistance to consumer criticism. A locally prestigious charitable organization uses prominent citizens to raise money to help blind people. Excluding other benefits, the fund-raising helps support the executive director's salary of $65,000 a year, while many of the agency's blind employees work for less than minimum wage.

GROUP PICKETS BIKING BENEFIT FOR THE BLIND

While more than 700 cyclists biked Sunday to benefit the Blind Association of Western New York, close to 80 informational pickets from the National Federation of the Blind walked to protest the association's policies.

"I'm not sure I understand," said John Shine, a cyclist from Norstar Bank. "My understanding was we were doing this for them."

And that is exactly why the pickets were there, they said, on the outskirts of the ninth annual bicycle "Ride in Plain Sight" to raise funds for the local Blind Association. The bicycle ride and a stationary bike challenge raised $47,553.50 for the association. Spokeswoman Joan Simon said that was a 42 percent increase over last year.

"We want the cyclists and the people of Western New York to know that there are people in the association workshops making $2.51 an hour while the executive director makes $65,000 a year," said Jennifer Vara of the Buffalo Chapter of the National Federation of the Blind of New York State and former resource center coordinator for the association.

"We don't think much of the money raised today will be used for the blind," she said. "Not when you have sighted workers being hired, and management and public relations consultants called in, and bonuses paid to management and a director with a car leased by the board."

Several guide dogs, sighted spouses, and friends walked with Federation of the Blind members, chanting and holding up posters with their claims against the association: "Backward philosophies, subminimum wages, contempt for the blind, threat of layoffs, decline in rehabilitation services, mismanagement, waste. . . ."

Federation members from Ohio, Pennsylvania, New Jersey, New York, and Maryland walked in the picket. Among them was James Gashel, government affairs director of the national group, the largest organization of the blind in America, who had come from its national headquarters in Baltimore. "The blind are being exploited here," he said. "They are working for next to nothing. They have no benefits, and this is supposed to be an association for the blind."

Vincent Taglairino, president of the Federation's Buffalo chapter, said "The (Blind Association) won't bargain with the union, which is only asking for minimum wage. The talks have been going on for a year. They're stalled at wages."

A year ago this week the nearly 70 employees in the sheltered workshops of the Blind Association became the first in the state, and one of only a few in the country, to unionize when they joined the Service Employees International Union.

"I'm among the fortunate ones," said Shirley Lazich of North Tonawanda, who has assembled expandable file folders in the workshop for the past six years. "I'm married and live mainly on my husband's wages. I couldn't live on mine."

Neither could Mike Deinhardt of Orchard Park, a co-worker in the shop for three years.

"Trying to make ends meet would be impossible," he said. "If it weren't for SSDI (Social Security Disability Insurance), I couldn't survive at all."

The association can legally pay less than the minimum wage of $4.25 per hour because sheltered workshop law allows it, said protesters who also criticized the association for "backward philosophies such as building apartments specifically for the blind when segregation based on a handicap is an old-fashioned idea that benefits no one."

"You can't please everybody," [said Ronald S. Maier, executive director of the association]. "We serve over 10,000 persons a year, of which this is a handful. We're not dismissing their concerns, but we wish they would work with us, not against us.

"Or against me. Some of them honestly and philosophically disagree with our policies. And some of them have a thing about me, rather than the agency. But we do satisfaction surveys, and they don't reflect any of this sort of negative feeling."

As for his salary, Maier said, "I don't pay myself, I don't hire myself. I am employed by the board."

"I guess everyone has a right to disagree," said Elizabeth C. Harvey, chairwoman of the Blind Association board of directors, "but I feel there are more constructive ways to disagree. Like positive suggestions. It's easier to be a critic than not."

Mrs. Harvey was unable to discuss salaries, she said, "because a contract is being negotiated."

As she spoke, 48 corporate teams of five persons each happily worked themselves into frenzies in the stationary bike challenge. Most of them appeared oblivious to onlookers and protesters. (Brandy, 1991, pp. 572–574)

Chapter 4

THE SOCIAL AND PSYCHOLOGICAL ASPECTS OF INTERACTION WITH BLIND PEOPLE

Rehabilitation interaction between the provider and the person served takes place in both institutional settings and the home. The expert is called in to deal with the client's problem. Unfortunately, the expert's experience "can lead him to form ideal conceptions of client interest, and this, together with professional standards of taste, efficiency, and farsightedness can sometimes conflict with what a particular client on a particular occasion considers to be his own best interests" (Goffman, 1961, p. 339).

Whether agreement or conflict results, the ideas and attitudes each party brings to the communication process facilitates or hinders the interaction. The setting of interaction, including the wider social context, often determines or greatly influences the interaction between persons with disabilities and others.

> The conceptualization of disability as deviance and reactions to this position [have] provide[d] the predominant framework for defining and interpreting disability. The consequences are enormous for the process dictates who shall be judged to be disabled and who shall control the definitional and treatment process. The identities and futures of persons with disabilities are forged by these processes so, as a result, much is at stake. On the institutional side, these interpretative processes define the group as a social problem and indicate which professionals and institutions are the appropriate agents of social control. According to the disability as deviance perspective, medicine, rehabilitation, and the government define and own the problem because they have authority in American society over [health] conditions and access to health care services. As a consequence, persons with disabilities have had their identities and futures defined for them. Not all persons with disabilities or even professionals, for that matter, are comfortable with this position because it usurps control from those individuals with the disabilities. (Albrecht, 1992, p. 77)

Impairments are the obvious basis of seeing disabilities as social problems. Individuals come forth to provide assistance which is often accepted, and relationships develop to facilitate the treatment or education process. "They were defined as a social problem by those in government, industry, [the] nascent rehabilitation field, and most importantly by the community of persons with disabilities and [the] general public, and, therefore, became [the] object of the emergent rehabilitation industry" (p. 78).

Physical disabilities, including blindness, are ascribed statuses (Friedson, 1965). Only in the most unusual cases do individuals choose blindness, for blind people are seldom happy about the situation. Still, it is my observation that they experience the full range of happiness or wellbeing that the population at large experiences. Under desirable conditions of education and rehabilitation, blindness becomes a nuisance to be managed. However, interaction between a blind person and those who would do him or her good frequently requires considerable management. "Many persons with disabilities are institutionalized within a discredited role and are trapped in relationships that feel far from 'normal' to them" (Albrecht, 1992, p. 74). From the point of view of blind persons, the most important thing is that they are as normal as others. However, from that of the helping individual, the overriding thing is the amount of vision. As Albrecht observed, "People who are disabled are often depersonalized in the disability business. In many discussions, impairments and disabilities are treated as objective conditions that exist in and of themselves. In this way, impairments and disabilities became reified, divorced from the individuals with the conditions and their readjusted sets of role relationships" (p. 70).

This chapter will focus on several different aspects of the rehabilitation process which frequently result in conflict or miscommunication. Experts, from physicians to counsellors, participate in the full array of stereotypes about blindness existing in a given culture. We will first examine interaction in the presence of a stigma or deformation of the body which attracts and holds our attention to the detriment of normal and routine communication (Goffman, 1963). Second, we will analyze images of the disabled person which emerge when the professional continually focuses on the disabling condition—the problem owned by the client—in the clinical or research setting. Beatris Wright calls this the fundamental negative bias. Third, we will review the consequences of these negative attitudes unwittingly held by providers of rehabilitation services and by those who conduct research about the special needs of blind people. Finally, we will evaluate the dominant paradigm widely held by professionals about the impact on blind people of the loss of visual contact with the environment. We will show the consequences of this model, including efforts to modify the environment or provide electronic alternatives to vision which, it is argued by many blind people, often result in greater dependence. The chapter concludes with three articles written by blind people in which we take a closer look at consumer response to their interaction with professionals.

Managing Spoiled Identity

Many observers have commented on the discomfort experienced when "normals" interact with people with disabilities. The attention of the "normal" person focuses on the discrediting, stigmatizing condition displayed by the disabled individual. As Goffman (1963) observed, "While the stranger is present before us, evidence can arise of his possessing an attribute that makes him different from others" (pp. 2–3). We may suddenly realize that the person has impaired vision, cannot hear, or is developmentally disabled to an extent hindering normal communication. Despite the stigma and the self-doubts of the disabled individual, the "normal" person will experience some strangeness in interacting with such people and in accepting them as essentially human. Others, however, will experience discomfort because they are uncertain and uninformed about how to treat the blind person. "As suggested, we are likely to give no open recognition to what is discrediting of him, and while this work of careful disattention is being done, the situation can become tense, uncertain, and ambiguous for all participants, especially the stigmatized one" (p. 41). When disabilities block normal, routine, "taken for granted" interaction, discomfort results for both parties.

Some blind persons are able to tolerate preoccupations others have with their success in dealing with blindness and respond in a manner which puts everyone at ease. Others, however become quite irritated. The problem is particularly difficult for blind people who have retained some degree of residual vision. Should they try to avoid the communication problem by trying to pass as sighted and risk greater problems if it fails? Or should they carry a white cane which will remove uncertainty, but, which will attract more attention to the stigmatizing condition? The organized blind movement has continually stressed a direct frontal approach to this problem in an attempt to change what it means to be blind. Television advertisements, radio spots, widely distributed brochures, films, books, seminars and publicized success stories have all been used to communicate that blind people are ordinary.

For example, in the nationally syndicated column of November 9, 1991, Ann Landers included guidelines for putting people at ease, which a reader had found in a brochure distributed by the National Federation of the Blind. To summarize, first, do not discuss the "wonderful compensations" of blindness; a blind person's other senses are not necessarily better, they are just more relied upon. Second, instead of grabbing a blind person's arm, let him or her suggest the form of contact to be made. Third, if you are curious, ask questions. Fourth, do not think of visually impaired people merely as "blind people." They are "people" who just happen to be visually impaired. Fifth, if you ask a question, ask the blind person, not the person he or she is with.

Managing communication and interaction is a continually recurring task for blind people because of the pervasiveness in most cultures of stereotypes about blindness. Not only are these stereotypes held by ordinary citizens, they are frequently reinforced and sometimes created by professionals who work with and study blind people.

The Fundamental Negative Bias

Beatris A. Wright (1988) analyzes what she calls the fundamental negative bias using examples taken from the work world of professionals in the field of rehabilitation. The fundamental bias results because the practitioner or researcher in the clinical or research setting is continually focused primarily on the disabling condition. The concentration of attention results in an overemphasis upon the stigmatizing condition at the expense of many "ordinary" or otherwise positive characteristics of the individual. For example, she presents the incident of a counselor seeking consultation from another professional on a fourteen-year-old delinquent youth. In describing this case the counselor listed ten negative qualities. Among the symptoms were assault, temper tantrums, stealing, car theft, arson, self destructive behavior (jumping out of a moving car), threats of harm to others, insatiable demands for attention, and under-achievement in school. The client was described as under-socialized and aggressive. When Wright then asked if the fourteen-year-old had anything going for him, the counselor mentioned that he had his own room in order, took care of his personal hygiene, liked to do things for others (although on his own terms), liked school, and had an IQ of 140. If not asked, the counselor probably would not have mentioned or even thought of these positive points.

Not only do rehabilitation workers often overlook positive qualities because of their preoccupation with negative features that become determinative in their perceptions, researchers do the same. They sometimes interpret findings as negative which ostensively are positive. Wright reviews a study that compared the interaction of able-bodied persons and confederate interviewers with and without apparent disabilities. Wright observes, "Although the major finding was that subjects consistently rated the interviewer with the disability more favorably on a variety of personality characteristics, the results were interpreted as supporting 'research indicating the operation of a sympathy effect to avoid the appearance of rejection or prejudice'" (pp. 4–5). The researcher then inferred that the person experiencing this effect would react negatively to sympathizers. Wright goes on to ask, "Was it not curious that the more positive evaluations of the handicapped interviewer, for example, more likeable, better attitude, should have been gratuitously interpreted as reflecting a negative sympathy effect?" She wonders why an alternative interpretation was not offered, namely that the subjects, upon recognizing the orthopedic disability, appreciated the success of the interviewer in meeting challenges, and accordingly recognized special positive qualities in the individual. This is neither phony nor disingenuous, says Wright (p. 5).

Wright's concept of the fundamental negative bias results from conditions in which something is observed or stands out as a dominant characteristic. If this characteristic is regarded as negative, and if such occurrences are infrequent, then the negative value ascribed to the object or person being observed is a major determiner of our perception of that individual. Wright's observations about the fundamental negative bias are similar to those of Goffman concerning the focus of the individual observer on the negative or intrusive characteristics of the person bearing a stigma. Negatively focused items frequently dominate attitude tests toward persons with disabilities and Wright considers this to be another manifestation of the fundamental negative bias. As she observed, using a disproportionate number of negative examples can have several undesirable consequences:

> We should be concerned that a preponderance of negatively worded items orienting thinking toward the negative side of possibilities strengthens a negative response bias. Also rejecting a negative statement is not the same affectively and cognitively as affirming a positive statement. Rejecting the idea, for example, that a particular group is often lazy or resentful does not

imply the opposite belief—that the group is often eager to work or appreciative. (p. 12)

The issue of the loading or frequent use of negative images is important because readers, students, and the informed public are usually ambivalent and their perceptions of groups with disabilities are likely to be unnecessarily influenced in a negative direction when the examples provided are negative. Positive examples are the primary means of changing public attitudes towards disabled persons, and these can generate positive attitudes and visions of opportunity within blind persons themselves. This is the reason frequently given for why the National Federation of the Blind uses the theme: "We are changing what it means to be blind" (p. 589).

This problem of negative imagery is most frequently apparent in the clinical setting, in research related to adjustments, or in the management of deficits. Negative attention is dominant in such settings, even though other resources such as peer support groups which provide positive images are also available. In the article cited above, Wright observes that one way to offset the power of the fundamental negative bias in problem oriented settings is for the clinician to keep in mind that it is more important to give as much attention to disclosing strengths and resources than to expose deficiencies and problems with respect to both the person and the environment.

> Their very nature is strongly influenced by these two vastly different orientations. Briefly, the succumbing framework highlights the difficulties of problems in terms of their devastating impact, not in terms of their challenge for meaningful adaptation. The emphasis is on the limitations of the person, the heartaches, suffering and tragedy. Such a state is viewed as pitiful and the person as an individual with a highly differentiated and unique personality is lost. (p. 14)

Negative Attitudes as a Source of Bias

In his presidential address to the 49th Annual Convention of the National Federation of the Blind, July 1989, President Marc Maurer stressed the importance of language to the future of the blind. One of the major purposes of the NFB is to change the meaning of blindness in this society. Images of blindness carried in our popular culture, obtained from advertising, humor, newspaper accounts and the like provide the symbols which prospective employers, new friends, or strangers use to guide their behavior toward, and treatment of, blind people. Maurer noted, "If the language is positive, our prospect will be correspondingly bright. If the words used to describe the condition of the blind are dismal, we will find that our chances for equality are equally bleak."

We have already noted the long history and pervasiveness of negative stereotypes about blindness and other disabilities. In addition to the folk or popular images of blindness existing in a society are those created by the intellectuals or experts who make careers out of studying the peculiar conditions of the blind. The failure of some scholars to be aware of or reflective about their own values and attitudes can influence their research and conclusions about blindness. Unfortunately, their individual reputations or their positions as researchers may give additional weight to the ideas which they spread to practitioners, the general public, and blind people. The issue is important because already existing negative imagery is reinforced and legitimated.

Symbols created by experts frequently guide or play a part in public policy decisions about programs for the blind. Scientific protocol, the creation of complex new constructs to further explain the problems of blind people, and the frequent use of mathematical manipulation of newly created data all lend heightened status to the image of blindness created by some professionals. To illustrate this problem we will review a recent work which purports to explain the self-esteem of blind people. In *Self-Esteem and Adjusting to Blindness,* Professor Dean Tuttle (1984) argues that there is a tendency for visually impaired persons to be more socially isolated, more socially immature, and more egocentric than sighted peers. As a result, blind people may also have a tendency to withdraw from family members who could provide the necessary support.

Tuttle's book attempts to interpret self-esteem and the development of the self of blind persons using a wide array of concepts from the history of developmental psychology, from William James to contemporary writers. He also analyzes problems encountered in adjusting to the trauma of blindness. Using trauma either as a medical or psychological concept, he describes it as a severe condition requiring significant intervention and often having lasting consequences. At four different places in the book, Professor Tuttle briefly mentions that no special psychological principles are necessary to understand blind people. However, while noting that personality traits are as variable among the visually impaired as among the sighted (p. 38), he goes on to write for 300 pages in which he describes the special and peculiar problems blind people encounter as they experience self-development and adjust to blindness. To support his arguments, Tuttle uses quotations from more than fifty biographical and autobiographical works of blind individuals. Because he is a social scientist, an educator in the field of blindness, and a blind person as well, one would think that he would present a fair balance and an evenhanded approach as he illustrates the peculiar and special situations of blind people. However, a closer look demonstrates only too well how a supposedly scientific and scholarly work can contribute unnecessarily to negative images about blindness. The unfortunate result, of course is an artificial and restricted picture of the world in which blind people are socialized.

When I first read Professor Tuttle's book, I was so struck by the pervasiveness of negative language about blindness that I re-read the text. Of his more than 250 quotations, fewer than twenty-five reflect positive images of blindness, another twenty could be called neutral, and approximately 200 are negative. For the most part, Tuttle selects only the dismal from what, for the most part, are success stories. "I got along the pavement as best I could—and that is another frightening experience difficult to describe to anyone who has not been blind, because though you are surrounded by noise, you have no coherent mental picture of what is around you. . . . I walked along in an enclosed gray little world a two-foot-square box of sounds around me" (p. 22). Another passage reads, "No other day in my life stands out quite so clearly or so horribly as the day on which I got the verdict. . . . His manner had kept full realization at bay until I was out in the street, then it struck with such force as to make it touch and go whether I did not go raving and screaming through the heart of Melbourne" (p. 161). A third reiterates Tuttle's theme: "A numbing terror fastened itself upon me when I was thus brought to realize that I was doomed to live the rest of my life in complete darkness. There was an agonizing feeling of helplessness and dismay at the thought of going through day after day without eyesight" (p. 175). I am not arguing that scholars must present only positive interpretations of blindness, although it would be refreshing. However, I am suggesting that the overwhelming preponderance of negative imagery reflects an unrecognized bias on the part of the author.

Despite the claim that he has assumed a sociological perspective on self-development, Dr. Tuttle completely ignores the influence of the organized blind on blind people in our society. In discussing significant others and reference groups, he advises that a blind person should be introduced to a teacher, school superintendent, counselor, or friend, and at one point he goes so far as to suggest that one meet another blind person to learn some practical strategies.

> However there is a time when the credibility of a message is much stronger coming from another blind person. The professional may want to arrange for a competent blind person to meet with the individual who is mourning. Areas of concern to be discussed with the recently blinded might include some "tricks of the trade" or some quickly and easily learned adaptive techniques. (pp. 179–180)

He does not suggest that it would be useful for a blind person to encounter groups of blind people who have positive images about blindness and who are committed to assisting themselves and others in the development of their human potential.

Robert Scott (1969) and Father Carroll (1961) made this same mistake of overlooking the organized blind in their major works about blindness. However, I would have hoped that by 1984 a specialist in the field of blindness such as Professor Tuttle would not have done so. He seems almost to go out of his way to applaud the influence of high tech gadgetry in the lives of blind people, but he seems ignorant of nationally distinguished leaders of the blind such as Dr. Jacobus tenBroek and Dr. Kenneth Jernigan or of countless hundreds of other people who have published successful stories of adaptation in the *Monitor* or other such periodicals. In fact, after he departs from the mainstream of literature about self development, he turns to a very narrow range of publication outlets, doubtlessly reinforcing his negative perspective.

Professor Tuttle (1986) reveals his attitude toward blindness in "Family Members Responding to a Visual Impairment." Here he illustrates what he calls the isolating factor of blindness, again from the same collection of biographical anecdotes. "I once knew a man who was afraid that because he happened not to see, he would be consigned to an eternity of loneliness where there would be nobody who would want to marry him" (p. 108). Tuttle is doubtless correct in reporting difficulties many blind people have experienced in adjusting to their situation. However, I have observed, talked with, and read about many hundreds of blind people from whom positive statements could be elicited. Professor Tuttle could have illustrated his ideas about adjustment using more positive imagery and made his argument with equal force.

How am I to explain the negative imagery that characterizes Professor Tuttle's work and the lack of attention to a major positive influence in the lives of many blind people? This book is just one more example of what appears to be the self-serving nature of much that passes for scientific research about blindness; it makes Professor Tuttle important as he speaks to seminars of professionals in the field of rehabilitation. It provides much additional imagery about what he thinks are the special and peculiar problems that blind people encounter and which require the exclusive attention and assistance of specially trained professionals. Professionals are needed in the education of blind persons, just as they are for anyone else, but they should, as a minimum requirement, be balanced in their attitudes towards blindness.

Psychologists are not the only disseminators of negative images about blindness. Physicians, including ophthalmologists who deal directly with vision, are often present at the most important occasions—when patients are informed about impending vision loss. Their attitudes towards blindness can be helpful or harmful to the degree that their advice influences the reactions and behavior of their patients. I have heard physicians and optometrists speak at conferences who demonstrated positive attitudes towards the future prospects of their patients. I have also heard prominent ophthalmologists say rehabilitation is not their concern. Perhaps the worst example of negative attitudes is reflected in an article by a physician, Dr. Stetten, published in the prestigious *New England Journal of Medicine* (1981). In this article he reviews his personal encounter with blindness and some of the resources he has used to manage his personal life. He mentions that as his vision deteriorated his "world [had] shrunk to a sphere with a radius of about an arm's length " (p. 458). He urges ophthalmologists to encourage their patients and to help them gain access to rehabilitation and other assistance. By so doing, physicians will earn the gratitude of the patient and "may transform the life of the blind from a living hell to a moderate inferno or, perhaps occasionally, a heaven" (p. 460). Dr. Stetten's intentions are laudable, but is such imagery about blindness helpful for the continuing education of professionals?

Dominant Paradigms about Blindness

In addition to the fundamental negative bias and the rather ordinary negative images about blindness frequently held by the general populous and by many rehabilitation workers, there are also dominant "theoretical" paradigms which have been developed to explain the problem of blindness and the kinds of specialized interventions which are required. Such assumptions about blindness result in architectural, engineering, and educational efforts intended to compensate for the absence of visual stimulation. Rehabilitation experts continue to experiment with technological modifications to the environment of blind people. Electronic canes, beeping subway train doors, and bells suspended over street crossings are ostensibly to enhance the safety and improve the mobility of blind persons.

Consumers usually argue that these "improvements" are too expensive, too specific to limited locations, technologically too complicated, and sometimes, simply a useless nuisance. These environmental adaptations, the blind argue, only increase dependency. Consumers who reject such improvements are sometimes considered recalcitrant, militant, or at best ungrateful and misinformed.

A deeper issue underlies the surface conflict between consumers and well-meaning rehabilitation experts. The sighted underestimate the amount of sensory information available to the blind. Thus, special arrangements are created, such as the beeping subway doors, which are thought to bring the blind into an improved relationship with the world as seen by the sighted. Each such effort makes the blind traveler less responsible for his or her life situations, removes decision making experiences, and undermines the ability of the blind to adequately process and understand the environment.

Brailling elevator buttons and hotel doors are examples of environmental adaptations which allow blind people to utilize their existing sensory abilities more efficiently. Computers with speech synthesizers and Braille printing capability exemplify electronic developments which enhance a blind person's ability to work and to interact with other people. Laptop Braille computers, including word processing software, greatly facilitates educational experiences for blind people. These examples are not intrusive and are no more expensive than similar work arrangements for other people. They do, however, promote occupational opportunities for blind people. Opposition to them only results when needless architectural and other expensive and complicated adaptations—which often promote dependency or heighten stereotypes—are erroneously called for, thus further hindering the integration of blind people into the wider community.

Underestimating natural alternatives to visual information has roots in historic images about blindness. Rehabilitation professionals have also been informed by a long series of articles and publications which stress that visual perception cannot be replaced. These arguments are best illustrated in the work of Dr. Berthold Lowenfeld, who published many articles in which he continually restated three limitations caused by blindness. First, the blind person is limited "in the range and variety of his concepts. . . . These limitations in the perceptual field cannot but result in a restriction of the range and variety of ideas and concepts in blind individuals" (p. 32). Second, the loss of vision impairs mobility. The blind person becomes "dependent upon the aid of others, thus afflicting his social relationships and attitudes in varying degrees" (p. 32). Third, without vision, the "isolating effect of this detachment restricts the blind individual in his or her control of the environment and results in increased feelings of insecurity and a state of higher nervous tension" (1944, p. 33). In short, Lowenfeld thought sight to be essential to carry on the normal activities of life.

Not only did he often restate these three themes, he was frequently cited by others, and being out of touch with reality came to be associated with scholarly writing about blindness. These three conditions may drive a blind person "into a world of unreality and fantasy" (p. 34). This idea was still appearing in the *Journal of Visual Impairment and Blindness* as recently as 1986 (Schuster). It is little wonder that many well-meaning professionals thought, and still think, that environments have to be modified to remedy deficits caused by the absence of visual stimulation. If one thinks a group of people are necessarily out of touch with reality, one can justify a wide array of programs and institutional arrangements. The frequently heated debate between those who would alter the environment to help the blind and those who reject such efforts seldom extends beyond the arguments mentioned above. Environmental adaption efforts are seldom analyzed and critiqued by rehabilitation professionals.

One notable exception is the recent contribution to the debate by Richard Mettler (1987) of the Nebraska Rehabilitation Services for the Visually Impaired. He states that if the experts were able to use abundant resources in their own way, the result would be a world of blind people living in a new kind of institution. It would not be a place of the sighted nor of the independent blind, but one of widespread environmental adaptation. In this institution the blind would not be encouraged to be competitive with the sighted in the real world of employment and independent living, but forced to operate in a special new world, arranged and managed by experts who would decide the new pathways by which the blind could approach but never enter the world of the sighted. According to Mettler, the medical model is not being supplemented, but is now being joined by the scientific/engineering model. Both focus on the individual blind person in whom the "problem" is located, and seek solutions based on the knowledge of "experts." Unfortunately, the autonomy of blind people is not a central element of the solutions available in either model. Instead, assumptions about the inherent limitations of blindness guide the development of arrangements intended to help the blind. For example, if it is thought that a blind person cannot travel independently, then stairwell barriers or special railings along sidewalks will be installed, thus depriving the blind person of responsibility and decision making.

Mettler has coined the term "neoinstitutionalization" to describe environmental arrangements that reduce the decision making occasions, thus increasing the dependency and diminishing the autonomy of blind persons. While evaluating environmental adaptations proposed for blind people, he observes that they possess sufficiently sound knowledge for managing their own environment:

> The first part establishes the fact that there is sound knowledge available for blind people to conceptualize and manage the physical environment on the basis of the reality of the world as known to them. The standard used in this model is the experience of a reasonable blind person trained in the skillful use of alternative (nonvisual) techniques, who possesses normal self-confidence and desire for self-direction, and who exercises care in his or her behavior. It is believed that strategies to modify the environment represent an attempt to substitute the legitimate concept formation of the blind by concepts grounded in a visual orientation to the world in the belief that there is no autonomous and reliable non-visual understanding of the world. (1987, p. 476)

He goes on to observe that typical environmental modifications reflect what may be best described as the "professional's conception of blindness." This has emerged from the general lay conception of blindness and has been enhanced, as we have indicated above, by a tradition of jargon developed by the professionals themselves. "The professional's conception considers blindness generally as a technical matter reducible to a series of difficulties in negotiating the physical environment because of the absence of normal vision" (p. 478). Mettler observes that the nature and extent of these difficulties are greatly exaggerated.

> The ability to move in the physical as well as the attitudinal environment has both personal and social value to blind people. The attitude that has led to typical environmental modification places control and responsibility for movement in the world outside the blind person and within control of the greater

society. This response runs counter to the most deeply held ideals of personal independence in our society. (pp. 480–481)

He also argues for considering the attitudinal impact of environmental adaptations on both the public in general and on blind people themselves.

Mettler analyzes environmental adaptations such as beeping traffic lights, which many consider critical as safety adaptations. Pedestrian walk lights do not signal to sighted pedestrians when it is safe to cross the street; they only tell which way to cross. Pedestrians still must act defensively to determine if motorists are obeying the law. Audible signals for the blind pedestrian do not provide any information the well-trained blind traveler cannot obtain by ordinary means. The normal auditory environment tells such a person not only whether the walk path is clear but also whether motorists are obeying the instructions of the traffic light. This vital information cannot be obtained from the beeping traffic light, and, in fact, may be obscured by the noise of the beeping traffic signals. "As it turns out, existing techniques skillfully executed by the user are the only ones that a blind traveler can use independently and safely" (p. 479).

However, since such devices are being used, it is important to consider how they affect the attitudinal environment.

> An unmistakable suggestion is given to the community at large, where audible traffic signals are in place, that blind people are profoundly out of touch with their surroundings and require a mechanical aid to be aware of their surroundings. Making traffic signals audible presumes that blind people lack judgement and skill sufficient for them to negotiate street crossings with traditional signals. . . . Almost any accommodative measure will exact some toll in the attitudinal environment, if only by reinforcing the public's tendency to interpret such devices as evidence that blind people as a class do not possess the abilities commonplace among sighted people. (p. 479)

Thus, because of audible traffic signals, not only will movement in the physical world not be enhanced for blind people, further damage will be done in the attitudinal world of the sighted. Will the blind person need environmental arrangements to find the desk chair, a water faucet or a handbag? Mettler also considers buzzers for subway car doors, which again provide nothing that blind people cannot learn by ordinary means.

> Environmental modification on behalf of blind people represents a new form of institutionalization, a tangible extension of a vestigial institutional mentality toward blindness in the greater society. This new form may properly be called neoinstitutionalization. The mind-set from which one provides physical,

social or political access to another is one of fairness and social justice. The mind-set from which one assumes responsibility for the safety and convenience of another is custodial, and of necessity must be supported by beliefs about a basic lack of ability in that other person. (p. 481)

In custodial arrangements much is done for the inmates and little is expected from them. The decisions of the institutions on behalf of the inmates are many and significant while little autonomy is delegated to the individual. At every turn control exists outside the individual. Residents are rewarded for behavior that reflects their incompetence and their willingness to adapt to the arbitrary institutional arrangements. Those who internalize these institutional arrangements as essential abandon prospects for becoming fully participating, self-determining adults.

No one has ever pretended that environmental modifications could be placed on a broad comprehensive scale throughout society. These occasional islands of environmental adaptation for the poorly trained blind individual are nothing more than a series of mini-institutions within the larger society. "From home to the local federal building and back, the blind person may feel at ease, for his convenience has been arranged by others, but this sense of security is hollow" (p. 481). Mettler concludes that environmental adaptations that have been designed to contribute to the social integration of blind people, in fact, have become additional barriers to their social integration and, in addition, have caused greater dependency. This entire process reinforces the notion that blind people are inherently incompetent, and: "the inescapable social consequence of this general belief is a reduction in opportunities for participation and success in most important areas of human endeavor" (p. 481). Clearly, there is a gap between the assumptions handicapped people make about themselves and the assumptions underlying many programs intended for their benefit. Just as clearly, these assumptions or environmental adaptations greatly affect interaction.

The gap between assumptions that clients make about themselves and the expectations of counselors is important to many clients. This gap can be documented. To counselors reading this paragraph, the issue may appear insignificant. However, it was an important issue to one group of fourteen students with whom I held a group discussion in September, 1992.

Federal regulations required that an individualized written rehabilitation program be developed reflecting agreement between counselor and student. One student, Jennifer Lehman, gave me permission to present examples from her Individualized Written Rehabilitation Program (IWRP) dated June 23, 1992, reflecting the input of her counselor from the Minnesota Department of Jobs and Training Services for the Blind and Visually Impaired. Miss Lehman's goal, according to her IWRP, was "to obtain a full adjustment to blindness program, subsequent higher education, and ultimate employment in social sciences as an instructor or other professional" (Minnesota Department of Jobs and Training Services for the Blind and Visually Impaired, p. 1). I now quote only two of the evaluation criteria suggested by her counselor in her agreement.

- Client will demonstrate and have documented, independent capability in all areas of orientation and mobility including demonstrated confidence in ability to learn new environments such as college campuses, offices, and unfamiliar communities at a 95% rate of success. (p. 2)
- Client will demonstrate and have documented, the full range of self care and homemaking capabilities involved in the general BLIND, Inc. program at 95% rate of success. (p. 3)

Another student from the same meeting reported an 85 percent success rate, suggested by her counselor.

As I mentioned earlier in this chapter, many professionals hold assumptions about the inherent limitations caused by blindness. Counselors subsequently develop ideas about the potential of clients which they communicate to clients. As indicated, these expectations can be described in terms of probability and can be incorporated in official documents. However, many students think that they, using alternative techniques, have the possibility of conducting daily living skills as well as anyone else. To Miss Lehman and her fellow students, her counselor's expectations were funny—but not too funny. I had asked this group of students, currently undergoing rehabilitation training, to tell me of experiences with the rehabilitation system which they found troublesome, harmful or objectionable. In this instance, the anticipated success rate was 85–95 percent (Minnesota is often considered a liberal state). The students considered this to be evidence of unfavorable counselor attitudes concerning the capability of blind people (see Chapter 8). Rather than having an agreement that the student would master the requisite skills, the counselor included language that he/she handles self-care and personal grooming skills only up to a certain level.

Discrimination is rooted in negative attitudes and stereotypes, and highly educated faculty of prestigious universities are not immune. Usually disguised as benevolence and laudatory comments about an applicant, the result is frequently discrimination based on beliefs about the limitations caused by blindness. I found no better illustration of this than in a series of letters reported by Jacobus tenBroek in the July 1967 issue of the *Braille Monitor.* These letters were communications between blind individuals and various officials of Stanford University. Despite the forcefulness of arguments, Stanford's final response came from an acting Dean because Dean Whitaker was on sabbatical and nothing could be done about the departmental decision.

BLINDNESS INSUPERABLE SAYS STANFORD

Editor's Note.—Frank Graff is a young, blind person who completed his undergraduate work at Cornell University at the end of the 1966–67 academic year. While still a senior, he applied for admission to do graduate work in history in a number of the country's best universities. One of these was Stanford University in Palo Alto, California. Stanford rejected Graff's application. The grounds given are remarkable for the mannerliness and kindliness of spirit, for their candor, and for their outright expression of discrimination based on blindness. Indeed, we have here a classic case of such discrimination complete with all the benevolent motives and mistaken impressions which lie at its foundation. Accordingly, we are reprinting, with only slight and irrelevant deletions, the letter of rejection sent by Stanford to Frank Graff and certain correspondence which ensued between Stanford University and Professor tenBroek. While all of this has been going on, Frank Graff has been accepted to do graduate work in a history department of another university of equal standing. Rejection of students by graduate schools and departments on grounds of blindness is surprisingly common. Many instances have come to light over the years including a number in recent years. The discriminatory element, however, is usually hidden behind a form letter turning down the application.

STANFORD UNIVERSITY
Stanford, California
ASSOCIATE PROVOST AND DEAN OF THE GRADUATE DIVISION

February 28, 1967

Mr. Frank Warren Graff
514 Wyckoff Road
Ithaca, New York 14850

Dear Mr. Graff:

I am sorry to have to tell you that the Department of History has recommended that you be denied admission to Stanford University for graduate work. I think that I can best indicate the Department's reason by quoting directly from the note on the report. "Mr. Graff is a young man of superior courage, and quite possibly superior intellect as well. But blindness in a research historian is virtually an insuperable handicap."

The basic problem, of course, is that graduate level involves scanning thousands of pages of material during research work, whereas that at the undergraduate level is more nearly confined to a reasonably manageable body of standard histories and monographs. Your experience as a student in undergraduate history courses is, therefore, not an accurate indication of the kind of problems that you will face as a graduate student.

I can assure you that the committee in the History Department took full account of your statement, including your explanation of how you intend to surmount your difficulties. I am very sorry indeed to disappoint you after what is undoubtedly a gallant achievement on your part, but those involved felt that in this case the kindest path was to prevent frustrations before they occurred, and I myself concur in their views.

Sincerely yours,

Virgil K. Whitaker

UNIVERSITY OF CALIFORNIA
DEPARTMENT OF POLITICAL SCIENCE
Berkeley, California

March 17, 1967

Professor Virgil K. Whitaker
Associate Provost and Dean of the Graduate Division
Stanford University
Stanford, California

Dear Professor Whitaker:

I hope you will not regard it amiss of me to intrude myself into a matter which you may think none of my business.

A young blind person named Frank Graff of Ithaca, New York, has been in touch with me about his rejection by the Stanford History Department as a graduate student. In your letter to him, you are frank to tell him that the grounds of the rejection are his blindness.

Graff got in touch with me because, though I am blind, I have been in the academic world for thirty years. He has consulted me about the problems of a blind person seeking to enter and to make his way in that profession. I have advised him that there is no reason why he can't do the work, including work in history.

Working with the use of readers undoubtedly presents some problems not experienced by an academician working with the use of his own eyes. The point you particularly mention—the ability to scan—is in some cases a good one. Lots of my seeing friends in the profession, however, can't scan either and proceed very much at a pace that I achieve. Indeed, by necessity the plodder may do more careful work.

In terms of production, I have been able to hold my own with most of my colleagues, having authored or co-authored four books and roughly fifty articles in the journals. Most of these have been in constitutional law and legal history. Nor do I rely solely on my own experience. There are literally dozens of blind persons teaching and researching in the colleges and universities of this country. I am personally acquainted with a good number of them. Some of them are productive; others not so much so, as in the case of our seeing colleagues. Productivity and competence to do research and writing are not, I am firmly convinced, functions of visual acuity, but of mental perceptiveness and habits of labor.

I know nothing about the extent to which Frank Graff possesses these latter qualities. Indeed, I would not only be content that you should apply your usual standards, but would insist that you do so. Exclusion on grounds of blindness alone, however, is, by everything that I know about blind people and about myself, altogether unwarranted—if you will permit me to say so.

I should be most happy to discuss this matter with you personally or, if you wish, to meet with a committee of your department. I urge you to reopen Graff's case and to decide it on its merits.

Cordially yours,

Jacobus tenBroek
Professor of Political Science

P.S. The sentiment expressed near the close of your letter, "... those involved felt that in this case the kindest path was to prevent frustrations before they occurred ...," rings a bell out of my past. One of the professors in a department where I had applied to be a teaching assistant argued that the application should be turned down so as not to "stir hopes that could not be fulfilled."

STANFORD UNIVERSITY
Stanford, California
ASSOCIATE PROVOST AND
DEAN OF THE GRADUATE DIVISION

March 21, 1967

Professor Jacobus tenBroek
Department of Political Science
University of California
Berkeley, California 94720

Dear Professor tenBroek:

I appreciate your thoughtful letter of March 17 about the application of Frank Graff to do graduate work in History at Stanford University. Since the decision was made by the Department of History, I am taking the liberty of forwarding your letter to that Department so that your testimony may be considered by the committee that made the original decision. Certainly you have written an eloquent letter.

Thank you again for your interest.

Sincerely yours,

Virgil K. Whitaker

cc: Professor David Potter

STANFORD UNIVERSITY
DEPARTMENT OF HISTORY
Stanford, California 94305

March 30, 1967

Professor Virgil Whitaker
Dean, The Graduate Division

Dear Professor Whitaker:

Thank you for sending us Professor tenBroek's letter concerning our negative action on the application of Frank Graff.

This is a complex matter, rendered more complex by the fact that the record includes letters of recommendation by referees, written opinions on the application by each member of the Admissions Committee, a report by the chairman of the committee to you, and your letter to Mr. Graff. None of these were identical, and the reasons for the action of the committee were not exclusively because of Mr. Graff's handicap. For instance, his most recent grades include more B's than A's, which is below the norm of the applicant whom we admit. We do believe, however, that an inability to glance through bodies of material is a substantial disadvantage to a man working in History and that it is more of a disadvantage in History than it would be in other academic fields.

In some ways Mr. tenBroek's own achievements, which we recognize and salute, are a proof of his own personal indominatability, and in no sense a reason for discounting the importance of the handicap.

In view of the full record, which, as we observe, did not turn entirely upon this one point, we do not feel that we can reopen the case. Perhaps Mr. tenBroek might be informed that our decision was not made solely on the issue of Mr. Graff's handicap.

Sincerely yours,

Lyman B. Van Slyke
Director of Graduate Admissions
Department of History

UNIVERSITY OF CALIFORNIA
DEPARTMENT OF POLITICAL SCIENCE
Berkeley, California

April 4, 1967

Dean Virgil K. Whitaker
The Graduate Division
Stanford University
Stanford, California

Dear Dean Whitaker:

. . . I hope you do not mind my returning to the subject of Frank Graff. Professor Van Slyke's letter makes it clear that the case will not be reopened. I am less concerned about that, however, than about the principle involved.

Professor Van Slyke indicates that factors other than blindness were given weight in the negative decision. Certainly I approve of applying to Graff whatever academic tests are used for everybody else. Professor Van Slyke's letter, however, only slightly changes the basis of discussion. That blindness was used as a factor at all is the critical matter not that it was the sole and exclusive ground of decision. The United States Supreme Court, for example, has said that race may not be invoked as an educational test at all, whatever the weight given to it in any individual case.

Professor Van Slyke argues that inability to scan bodies of material is a substantial disadvantage in history, and that it is more of a disadvantage in that field than in others. I concede the first point, but doubt the second. Vast bodies of material must be covered in all the social sciences. In law, the reading is particularly heavy. Even though one is not doing legal research, the practitioner, the professor, and the judge all must keep abreast of the work of innumerable courts, and success in any given lawsuit may well depend upon research competence. Yet there are somewhere between one and two hundred blind persons practicing law in the United States—at least a dozen judges from trial courts to the Supreme Court and a handful or more teachers and scholars. So, even though we would admit the disadvantage of inability to scan, it does not follow that this is such a disadvantage as should or does rule blind persons out of the research profession.

What is even more critical, in my point of view, than the fact that the department decision rests on preconceptions about blindness rather than on actual knowledge, is the fact that a test is applied to Graff which is not applied to other applicants. The history department, I am sure, does not examine students in terms of their ability to scan when it admits them. To my certain knowledge there are lots of professors in the social sciences on the Berkeley campus who have a very poor ability to scan, and some of these are in our history department. The same surely must be true of graduate students here and elsewhere.

If in a meeting of a department in the social sciences or in history a faculty member should propose to establish a scanning test for all graduate student admissions, I think you would be opposed to it on general grounds. The question really isn't can a student scan; it is can he do the work, and this is dominantly a question of intellectual capacity. If he actually produces, who cares what his methods are? But in the absence of a department's adopting any such test to be applied to all students, there can be no justification whatsoever for applying it to particular students, and especially for selecting the students to whom it is to be applied on the basis of general misimpressions about the nature of blindness and its limitations.

I am flattered by Professor Van Slyke's characterization of me as personally indomitable. This is a mode of argument which has always plagued the task of opening employment opportunities for blind people. First, the prospective employer says that it may be possible for blind persons to work in somebody else's field, but not in mine. Then he explains away successful blind people in his field by pointing to their unusual qualities. As a matter of fact, as I have pointed out before, blind people have succeeded and do succeed as teachers and scholars in history, in other social sciences, in law, and in many more fabulous fields. A blind person of my acquaintance, over the disbelief and resistance of the faculty, took a Ph.D. in chemistry and is now a research chemist. Another blind person of my acquaintance did the same in nuclear physics. The argument is always the same; it may be that they can succeed somewhere else. What is overlooked in using the argument about exceptional blind persons is the number of them there are and the variety of fields in which they have succeeded. But, in addition, if successful blind persons are to be explained away in terms of their particular qualities, would it not make sense for the prospective employer to test for those qualities in the newly appearing blind persons? For example, does the Stanford History Department have any reason to suppose that Frank Graff is not "personally indomitable?" First they require him to be able to scan; then they require him to be personally indomitable. If he cannot do one and is not the other, then he may not be a graduate student in history, even though other students are admitted who cannot scan and are not personally indomitable.

Truly, the handicap of blindness lies not so much in the physical fact as in the misconceptions of sighted people about it and the exclusionary actions which they take on the basis of those misconceptions.

Yours sincerely,

Jacobus tenBroek (pp. 402–409)

Another issue which currently attracts much interest in professional literature about blindness is the correct word to describe loss of vision — the "B" word should be avoided whenever possible. It is preferable to use "partially sighted," "limited vision," "low vision," "persons who are blind," and so forth rather than "blind persons." "Persons who are blind" is used because kind people want to focus on the person and not the characteristic of blindness. However, when we use adjectives positively we speak of intelligent people, beautiful people, or confident people. The philosophy of the NFB is to remove the idea of shame or untouchability from the word "blind." It is all right to be a blind person.

The insistence of clinics, professionals, and editors of journals upon using "people with blindness" or "persons with disabilities" unintentionally perpetuates the negative imagery. The issue is more than semantic, as Jim Omvig illustrated in the July 1983 *Braille Monitor.*

ARE WE BLIND, OR SOMETHING ELSE?
WHAT'S IN A WORD?

In the March 1983 *Monitor* we reprinted a speech which I delivered at our Michigan convention on what a commission for the blind should be. There have been quite a number of comments about it and reactions to it. Among others, I received a letter from Larry Israel, President, Visualtec regarding our use of the word "blind." Since the issue is one which frequently comes up, it seemed to me that a very thorough response was in order. Following is a complete reprint of Mr. Israel's letter together with my reply:

Santa Monica, California
March 21, 1983

Dear Mr. Omvig,

I enjoyed the reprint of your address which appeared in *The Braille Monitor* under the title "What We Can Expect From a Commission for the Blind: Viewpoint From the Consumers."

Although much of what you said was not unfamiliar to me, since I have been involved with blindness, NFB, etc., for nearly twelve years, there are a few comments you made about which I'd like to open some sort of discussion with you or other knowledgeable people associated with NFB.

As you may know, Visualtec is concerned solely with the provision of electronic visual aids (machines, if you prefer that terminology) for people who have severe visual limitations, but are not totally blind. We have no bias against the totally blind—it just happens that we don't serve that community. Because of this environment, issues and terminology related to blindness other than total blindness are of particular interest to us.

The major item in your talk which triggers a response is under the bold-face heading: "Blindness must be discussed and the word 'blind' must be used and stressed." The last sentence in the paragraph then says: "Therefore, such phrases as 'visually impaired, visually limited, or sightless' should not be used."

Setting aside the fact that "sightless" may not be in the same category as the first two phrases, would I be correct in assuming that this sentence should be qualified by adding: " . . . to describe persons totally without sight," or did you intend it to stand unqualified? If the latter, how do you fairly and accurately describe persons who have visual impairments or limitation, but are not totally blind? How is Visualtek to describe, in literature and elsewhere, the type of persons it is able to serve, if we should not use such terminology?

We have always used the terms "visually impaired" and "visually limited" to mean someone who had an impairment or limitation, but was not totally without light perception (or so close to it such that any distinction was meaningless). We know how to use the word "blind," but we tend to say "totally blind" merely to ensure clear communication. Over the years, we have found that the word "blind" is not well-defined; many people continue to think that "blind" means "totally without sight."

I could reasonably put the issue in this way: wouldn't you agree that there are many situations where it is desirable to clearly communicate whether a person was totally without light perception, or had usable but severely limited visual capabilities? Clearly, we could develop lengthier descriptions which would communicate such distinctions clearly, but the history of human communication has been to develop shorthand modes of communication in many areas. I would submit that is what most people mean by "visually impaired" or "visually limited." I'm not condoning . . . and in fact would criticize . . . use of such terms as euphemisms for blind. I share your beliefs in dealing openly and straightforwardly with blindness, and using the word "blind" when it is appropriate.

If I am wrong, and there is in fact widespread and damaging use of "visually impaired" and "visually limited" to conceal the truth of blindness, then what would you suggest as convenient and acceptable ways to draw the distinction, when it is desirable or necessary to do so?

What does "blind" mean? I am familiar with the legal definition, but it seems useful only in a legal domain, or as an arbitrary classifier. Sam Genensky, whose work you are probably familiar with, has attempted to establish a series of terms to describe different levels of functional capability, which span the spectrum from total blindness to those whose visual impairment does not even qualify them as legally blind. Although there seems to be merit in his attempts to improve communications on this topic, I do not believe his definitions are widely understood, nor have they been widely accepted, to the best of my knowledge.

Has NFB ever addressed this question, whether formally or informally? Can you provide me with a definition of blindness which helps to unmuddy the waters, yet is not arbitrary or overly technical?

To get a bit more specific (by way of example), how would you describe and propose dealing with a person whose visual capabilities permitted adequate mobility without assistance, and no significant problems regarding orientation, yet couldn't read worth a damn using even the best correction available. Describing such a person as "blind" is misleading at best, and certainly is no aid to clear communications (although there may be some situations where it is adequate or tolerable to use that description). It would not seem necessary or desirable, in most cases, for such a person to be at the kind of center you describe. I might note that there appear to be substantial numbers of people, who can be described in this manner, who are active and energetic members of NFB. One would hardly know it, from reading your literature!

Please be assured that this letter comes to you in a spirit of honest and open inquiry. I have learned much, over the past 12 years, from reading *The Braille Monitor.* If this letter helps me to learn more, it will be well worth the effort.

Sincerely,

Larry Israel,
President, Visualtek

––––––––––

Baltimore, Maryland
April 8, 1983

Dear Mr. Israel:

This will thank you for and reply to your letter of March 21, 1983, concerning the use of the word "blind" as discussed in our March reprint of my speech, "What We Can Expect From a Commission for the Blind, Viewpoint From the Consumers." I very much appreciate the fact that you are a regular *Monitor* reader, that the speech interested you and that you were willing to take the time to write. (Incidentally, I have also reviewed letters which you have written on this subject to Mrs. Pat Munson of the NFB, Western Division.)

Let me begin with a very general observation which may appear to be unrelated to the questions you raise but which, I assure you, is key as we of the Federation work to improve the quality of life for all blind persons. If more professionals would make a sincere effort as you have to learn and understand the philosophies and goals of the National Federation of the Blind rather than simply to go on the attack concerning what they do not understand, there would be much more harmony and goodwill, and the world would be a better place for all blind persons. I commend you for concluding your letter by saying "If this letter helps me to learn more, it will be well worth the effort," and I hope you mean what you say.

Now, let us turn to your letter. First, you are right on target in that the legal definitions of blindness don't help much—at best, they give only loose guidance. While most persons who are "legally blind" cannot function well with regular sized inkprint, some really do function efficiently and for sustained periods of time. On the other hand, there are some persons who are not "legally blind" who can scarcely function at all using inkprint. And so it goes with all facets of human endeavor. Then, there are some persons, totally blind, legally blind or not legally blind who do not function at all well with sighted techniques. However, they insist upon using them no matter how ineffective they may be and steadfastly refuse to use "blind" techniques even though such techniques would be far superior to sighted techniques.

Since it would be difficult to answer your letter question by question, I shall first provide you with a general response and statement. Then, if questions remain, I shall answer them individually.

The basic question you raise is this: When either I as an individual or the National Federation of the Blind use the word "blind," are we talking only about those who are totally blind or do we also intend to include and describe those persons who have some remaining vision which is quite usable at least in some situations?

Those of us who have a profound interest in improving the quality of life for all blind persons have given serious and extensive thought as to just how this goal can best be achieved. It did not take too long to conclude that nothing else we can do really matters very much if we are not willing first to face the "real" issue and to overcome it: namely, how do we perceive ourselves, and how are we perceived by others around us?

I believe that this simple analogy will help you to understand: Black persons in our country are a minority with every negative connotation which the word "minority" implies. They are stereotyped; they have faced and continue to face terrible discrimination; and their problem is clearly a social one, an attitudinal one, not a physical one. Obviously, the color of one's skin has nothing whatever to do with basic normality or anything to do with a person's right to enjoy equal opportunity. But, because of prejudice and misconception, black persons have been thought of (and have thought of themselves) as being all alike, inferior, lacking in ability, abnormal, unequal and literally as a people not entitled to the rights and privileges which go hand in hand with first-class citizenship.

Through the years black persons have taken two separate and very diverse approaches in an effort to solve their problems. I am sure I don't need to remind you that there were some (sadly, far too many) who thought that they could solve their problems by pretending that they were white (normal). They rubbed a variety of potions on their skin to lighten its color and straightened their hair if it happened to be curly. But, this didn't change a thing—no one was fooled, particularly the black person who was so ashamed of being black that he or she actually played out the deception. What a life! How would it feel to "pass off" for white fearing all the while that someone would find out?

Thank God for enlightened black leaders: leaders who said, "It's o.k. to be black; it's respectable to be black; it's normal to be black; and, rather than trying to solve our problem by pretending we are white, if we have any sense, we will get together and change social attitudes so that it is respectable to be black; and the first step is for 'us' to teach ourselves new attitudes." With this kind of positive, social thinking, change began!

But, what of those who are only "partially black," or is it "partially white"—those who are the offspring of mixed marriages? Are they black or are they white or are they something else altogether? Rightly or wrongly, people in our country both black and white, regard these individuals as black. Because of prejudice and discrimination, they face the same problems which are faced by the "totally black," and they must take the same steps if they intend to solve their problems. Can you imagine such an individual, faced either with problems of discrimination or a lack of self esteem, saying, "Why, I'm not black, I'm mulatto."

Now, let us return to those of us who are blind, whether we are totally blind or have some usable vision. Our problem is precisely the same as that of black persons; we are a minority; we are stereotyped; we have faced and continue to face terrible discrimination; and "our" problem is clearly a social one, an attitudinal one, not a physical one. Obviously, the amount of vision in one's eyes has nothing whatever to do with basic normality and competency, and it should have nothing to do with a person's right to enjoy equal opportunity. But, because of prejudice and misconception, blind persons have been thought of (and have thought of themselves) as being all alike, inferior, lacking in ability, abnormal, unequal and literally as a people not entitled to the rights and privileges which go hand in hand with first-class citizenship.

As with blacks, it follows from this type of negative social thinking and from long-standing social conditioning that blind persons have gone through a period of feeling shame and embarrassment. Who wants to be an inferior? Why not just pretend you are sighted—refuse to use Braille, refuse to use a long cane or dog guide, refuse to put your hands on something to "see" it, or refuse to let anyone know that you are blind?

Ah, what a solution! All we really do is provide more income for the medical profession for treating ulcers or psychological problems.

What is the difference if an employer or school refuses to hire you or let you in, "because you are blind," "because you are sightless," "because you are visually impaired" or "just because you are a little hard of seeing"? There is no difference! The problems, the results and the solutions are the same no matter what you call yourself or what you are called by others—A ROSE, IS A ROSE, IS A ROSE.

We of the Federation have taken a lesson from black persons, and we do not intend to make the same mistake which was made by some of them. We intend to work together towards the day when blind people have true equality, when it is respectable to be blind and when we can say, as the author said, "I'm o.k., you're o.k." The very first step in this process is for those of us who are blind to "accept" rather than deny our blindness, to come to have a real belief in ourselves and then to work together to change broader social thinking so that fear and shame may be replaced with confidence, hope and opportunity.

The Federation's course is clear and well charted. The only question which remains is whether blind persons not in the Federation, agencies and service providers, and manufacturers of technology can grasp the importance of changing the image of what it means to be blind, and will join with us to do something about it.

In your letter you asked whether anyone has ever developed a workable definition of blindness. Yes! We have! Quite a number of years ago our national President, Dr. Kenneth Jernigan, wrote a paper entitled "A Definition of Blindness" (copy attached). We of the Federation have incorporated this document into our overall philosophy, and I hope that you will study it thoroughly and do likewise. Dr. Jernigan states in part as follows:

> One is blind to the extent that he must devise alternative techniques to do efficiently those things which he would do with sight if he had normal vision. An individual may properly be said to be "blind" or a "blind person" when he has to devise so many alternative techniques—that is, if he is to function efficiently—that his pattern of daily living is substantially altered. . . .
>
> I repeat that, in my opinion, blindness can best be defined not physically or medically but functionally or sociologically. The alternative techniques which must be learned are the same for those born blind as for those who become blind as adults. They are quite similar (or should be) for those who are totally blind or nearly so and those who are "partially sighted" and yet are blind in the terms of the usually accepted legal definition. In other words, I believe that the complex distinctions which are often made between those who have partial sight and those who are totally blind, between those who have been blind from childhood and those who have become blind as adults are largely meaningless. In fact, they are often harmful since they place the wrong emphasis on blindness and its problems. Perhaps the greatest danger in the field of work for the blind today is the tendency to be hypnotized by jargon.

Finally, on philosophy, add the following: Blind people are normal people who, with proper training and opportunity and through the use of alternative techniques including effective low vision aids, can participate fully and successfully in the total range of human endeavor. However, a very real danger exists when blind persons deny their blindness and use sighted techniques which, for them are inferior to blind techniques. Such an individual will most likely fail, but it is not because of his or her blindness—it is because of a denial of blindness and the resulting inability to function.

So where does all of this leave you, Visualtek, rehabilitation and other professionals in the field? Since it can hardly be said that you are selling your equipment to "sighted persons," why not sell it to blind persons who have visual capabilities in certain situations? I assume that you would not believe that the Federation would approach an employer about hiring a blind person with some vision and decline to tell that employer that the individual has some vision which may be useful for some things. Contrary to what some of our antagonists preach, we are not "making blind people" out of sighted people.

Turning to rehabilitation, in your letter you say, "It would not seem necessary or desirable, in most cases, for such a person [having some vision] to be at the kind of center you describe." If you will reread my speech, you will find quite a long discussion on the use of sleepshades in an orientation center for those blind students who have some vision so that they can properly learn alternative techniques and also become competent to make a decision as to whether, for efficiency, they should use either blind or sighted techniques.

The word "blind" should also be used in education, and blind children should be taught to read and write Braille, cane travel, etcetera. Again, those of us who have considerable experience in this field are shocked and dismayed when we see Braille training being denied blind children who can read either through large print or visual aids at no more than fifteen or twenty words a minute. Apparently it has not occurred to the teachers and professionals that such deprivation will hurt the blind child for the rest of his or her life.

Again, I appreciate the fact that you have written to me. Because of the importance of this issue, I have taken more than a little time to respond. I hope that you will make a thorough study of this information and that it is helpful to you.

Very truly yours,

James H. Omvig

P.S. To make sure that this letter is not confusing to you, let me make it very clear that we are not saying and have never said that a device such as the Visualtek cannot be a valuable tool for a blind person. It can be if we know when to use it and when not to. (pp. 227–232)

In this chapter I have noted the negative imagery about blindness unwittingly held by many professionals and the failure of some counselors to use peer support groups for blind individuals receiving rehabilitation services. Probably nothing is more important in changing the self-image of a blind person than positive role models. All of this is illustrated by the experience of Katherine Horn Randall (1989) as she describes the time she spent in a residential rehabilitation program.

In February of 1979 I took the train to Chicago to learn to function as a blind person at the Illinois Visually Handicapped Institution (IVHI), the state training center for blind and newly blind adults. I would not learn about and join the National Federation of the Blind for another three long years. No one at IVHI told me that the Federation had a Chicago chapter where I could meet other blind people.

My confidence was at rock bottom. I knew that to restore it I must learn to use Braille and the white cane. But I also had my own built-in positive attitude and philosophy that blindness was not going to change my life style or destroy my zest for living.

I would need every bit of determination I had to face the months to come. I now realize that an administrative and teaching staff without a positive approach to blindness and deep-seated belief in blind people cannot possibly teach the skills of blindness well enough for their students to use them competitively in the real world.

An atmosphere of hopelessness and eternal despair hit me as I entered the lobby. Students were sitting aimlessly around with nothing to do and nowhere to go.

In fact, until I had lived at IVHI for a while, I didn't know that I could be a rebel when necessary. I battled with the administrative staff to stop treating adults who happen to be blind like three-year-olds. We forced administrators to stop wasting time in weekly general gripe sessions that we called "Hee Haw," at least for the semester I was there.

I was required to attend group therapy sessions that wasted my time. I told the psychologist that I would not be returning to these meetings. I was blind, not mentally ill.

Assignments were seldom given, so evenings and weekends were long. I worked on Braille and spent more time than is healthy bar-hopping, trying to relieve the awful tension IVHI created inside me.

We students talked late into the night about our blindness and how we hoped to put the pieces of our lives together when we went home. We needed positive blind role-models to emulate, and we didn't have them. If I could have met Chicago Chapter members of the NFB,

I would have had people to turn to who were blind and were truly making it in the real world. With friends as legitimate role models I would have demanded more of IVHI and more of myself.

The six years I have spent as a Federationist have tremendously changed and enhanced my life. I now have hundreds of blind friends from all over the United States who serve as excellent role models for me and for other people who happen to be blind. My Federation work helps me to succeed as a city alderman today. I serve as Jacksonville Theatre Guild President and as Vice President of the MacMurray College Alumni Board. I have more Federation and community work to do each day than I can possibly accomplish, and I have never been happier in my life.

The Federation gave me back my self-respect as a blind person, and that is a gift beyond all measure. (p. 466)

We have argued that a dominant idea about blindness concerns the irreplaceable loss of vision. The result has been almost endless efforts, usually at great public expense, to alter the environment experienced by blind people. This results in removal of decision making and responsibility from the individual blind person and heightens the already negative attitudes about special arrangements that employers and the public make to accommodate blind people. The following two articles, from among at least thirty I could have included, illustrate the basis of consumer rejection of arrangements which are both costly and promote unnecessary dependency.

ELECTRONIC CANES BRING PROTEST FROM THE BLIND

(Note: This article is taken from the December, 1983, issue of *Que Pasa*, the newsletter of the National Federation of the Blind of New Mexico.)

For the past two years, Dr. Wolfgang Prieser from the University of New Mexico has been working on the development of an electronic guidance system for the blind. A prototype of Dr. Prieser's guidance system has been installed on the second floor of the Student Union Building, and it is anticipated that the device will eventually be installed throughout the University campus.

On the surface, the device seems harmless enough. Wires are run under the floor for the purpose of transmitting a signal to an electronic cane. The cane acts as a receiver, beeping as long as it stays close over the wire.

When the device was originally field tested, the blind spoke out against it from both a philosophical and practical perspective. First, the device assumes that conventional mobility techniques do not allow the blind to travel with true independence. The premise on which the device is based is false as demonstrated by the thousands of blind men and women who travel independently each day. The device seeks to solve a problem which the blind do not have. Given proper training, a blind person can travel with confidence wherever he or she cares to go.

Second, the device seems impractical at best. Its only conceivable merit is for a blind person who only has to go from one given point to another without variation. If, for example, a blind person wished only to travel from the door of the Student Union Building to the lunch counter and back, then the device might work. However, we know of no blind person whose travel is that predictable and routinized. Therefore, it seems that the device is limiting to the travel of the blind.

At one point there was talk of making the device more versatile by means of running several wires each transmitting a different tone. One tone would take you to the snack bar, another to an administrative office, another to the elevator, and so on. It is hard to take seriously this proposal as an innovation. Rather than making the device more versatile, the developer would make it necessary for a lengthy training process to accompany use of the device, not to mention the inherent problem for those of us who cannot easily distinguish a particular tone or pitch.

Nevertheless, Dr. Prieser persists in promoting his device as a breakthrough for the blind. When faced with opposition from the blind, Dr. Prieser assumed a curious point of view. Recently Dr. Prieser was presented with a copy of Federation Resolution 83-03, which was unanimously adopted at our state convention last April. The resolution expresses the opposition of the blind to the electronic guidance system project. During an interview on KUMN Radio, which was broadcast December 9, 1983, Dr. Prieser defended his project by saying that the guidance system may eventually be used by the public at large and only secondarily by the blind. He suggests that the guidance system may be helpful to a sighted person as he or she hurries down a smoke filled corridor in a hotel fire. Surely Dr. Prieser cannot seriously believe that in just a few years guests checking into a Hilton

Hotel will be issued, in addition to a key, an electronic cane for use in case of a fire. Perhaps each guest will have a bellman who will provide instruction in the use of the cane. Far-fetched? We believe so.

Of greater concern than the impracticality of the guidance system is the effect it has on public attitudes toward the blind. On Friday, November 18, 1983, Dave Nordstrand wrote an article which appeared in the *Albuquerque Tribune* praising the electronic guidance system as a breakthrough for the blind. Why did Mr. Nordstrand praise the guidance system? The article made clear that Mr. Nordstrand holds as true some of the most demeaning stereotypes about blindness and therefore accepts the premise on which the guidance system is based. That is, that the blind are incapable of finding their way independently and therefore must be aided in getting from place to place.

Our state president, Fred Schroeder, wrote to Dr. Prieser to explain our opposition to the guidance system and why we feel that prejudicial attitudes such as Mr. Nordstrand's are only perpetuated by its existence. President Schroeder's letter follows in its entirety:

Dr. Wolfgang Prieser
Department of Architecture and Planning
University of New Mexico

Dear Dr. Prieser:

I am writing concerning the electronic guidance system which you designed for use by blind students on the University of New Mexico campus. It is my understanding that this system has been installed on the second floor of the Student Union Building and that plans are underway to expand the system to other areas of the campus.

Let me begin by saying that the National Federation of the Blind of New Mexico is the largest organization of blind people in the state. Our members include the very young, as well as the very old, those with advanced academic qualifications and those with little formal education, the employed and the unemployed, the newly blinded, and those who have been blind since birth. In short, we represent the broadest possible cross section of society and are joined together by the common characteristic of blindness. We have been organized since 1956 and have been instrumental in effecting social change to improve the quality of life for the blind. We are responsible for the introduction and passage of the New Mexico White Cane Law, as well as legislation creating an orientation center in Alamogordo, which provides rehabilitation training to the blind of the state. We currently operate an aggressive program known as Job Opportunities for the Blind (JOB), which has been instrumental in helping many blind New Mexicans obtain meaningful employment. All of our programs and activities are carried out entirely by the volunteer efforts of our members. We have no paid staff on which to rely. In concept and in practice the National Federation of the Blind of New Mexico is not an organization speaking for the blind—it is the blind speaking for themselves.

Fundamental to the progress which the blind have made is the ability to adapt ourselves to the world as it is. Part of this process is acquiring the skill of reading Braille as an alternative to print and learning to use a long white cane or dog guide as an alternative to using visual cues when traveling. With adequate training and opportunity we are able to compete on a basis of equality with the sighted. For this reason, we are firmly committed to ensuring that the blind have ready access to good rehabilitation training and to educating the public as to the abilities of the blind.

We have found that given proper travel training a blind person can travel easily and confidently in both familiar and unfamiliar surroundings. Airports, shopping centers, and even a university setting pose no particular difficulty with which the well-trained traveler cannot easily cope. If a blind person is having difficulty in traveling around the University of New Mexico campus, then there is clearly a need for additional travel training, not a special electronic travel aid.

The guidance system which you have had installed on the second floor of the Student Union Building poses a limitation to independent travel rather than an opening of new freedom of movement for the blind. If a blind person truly needed the aid which your electronic guidance system offers, then the blind person would be restricted to traveling independently on one floor of one building on campus. Since the special canes which accompany the guidance system are only available through the Special Services Office, the practicality of an electronic guidance system must be questioned. After all, if a blind person can get from his or her home to the Special Services Office to pick up the special cane and next to the second floor of the Student

Union where the guidance system is available, then one is prompted to question whether the special guidance system is truly necessary to the blind person's ability to travel. You may argue that the guidance system, in its present form, is only the beginning and that some day the system will be expanded throughout the campus and perhaps even out into the community at large. Financial implications not withstanding, it is difficult to conceive of a guidance system which will give the blind more freedom than is already readily available.

Nevertheless, the fundamental problem with an electronic guidance system is the philosophical premise upon which it is based. The underlying attitude behind its creation stems from an image of the hopeless, helpless blind groping their way timidly through a world fraught with danger and uncertainty. The electronic guidance system presumes that the blind are incapable of finding their way and therefore must be aided by an elaborate, electronic custodian. In an article entitled "Visionary UNM Project Eyes New Hope for the Blind," which appeared in the *Albuquerque Tribune* on Friday, November 18, 1983, Dave Nordstrand describes his experience while wearing a blindfold as traveling, "pinball fashion, spinning, bouncing off walls, cursing, losing my balance, and all the while fearing I was going to drop off the edge of the universe." On the basis of this distorted and deplorably demeaning image of blindness, Mr. Nordstrand applauds the electronic guidance system as means of sparing the blind from the terror of traveling through a hostile environment. The National Federation of the Blind has devoted itself to improving the public image of blindness and to tearing down the age-old attitudes which are based on a conception of blindness as representing an incapacity to function normally in society. By installing an electronic guidance system the public is reinforced in its belief that the blind are unable to travel without elaborate accommodation. The effect of this attitude is to limit social and economic opportunities for the blind. An employer, knowing of your electronic guidance system, would most certainly be reticent to employ a blind person because it would be presumed that the place of employment would first require extensive and costly modification, that is, the installation of a similar guidance system before a blind person could function on the job. The guidance system which you view as an enhancement to a blind person's ability to travel translates into lost opportunities and social isolation. The blind are not plagued with architectural barriers but rather attitudinal barriers. Our success in improving social and economic conditions for the blind has come from our ability to adapt ourselves to the world rather than relying on the benevolence of the world to adapt to us. This basic philosophy is reminiscent of the parable which poses the question, whether it is better to give a starving man a fish or to teach him how to catch fish for himself.

Please understand the depth of feeling behind our position. As blind people we seek to live normal lives as fully participating, contributing members of society. We do not seek elaborate accommodations from the public, but simply an understanding of the true meaning of blindness. We recognize that you are not responsible for the insulting condescension of Mr. Nordstrand's recent article but simply urge you to understand that your electronic guidance system will inevitably result in the reinforcement and proliferation of attitudes such as the ones expressed by Mr. Nordstrand. I am enclosing a copy of Resolution 83-03, which was unanimously adopted at the annual convention of the National Federation of the Blind of New Mexico.

If I can provide additional information which will help to clarify our position, please do not hesitate to contact me.

Very truly yours,

Fred Schroeder, President
National Federation of the Blind of
New Mexico

As blind people we have difficulty in understanding why the public persists in promoting projects for our benefit which we do not need and do not want. There are many technological developments which are useful to the blind, such as talking computers, compact tape recorders, and talking calculators. Our opposition is not to technology but rather to the development of programs and devices which are founded on conceptions of blindness which draw their definition from myth and tradition. Together we can plot a course rich with the promise of true progress toward securing equality for the blind. (Jernigan, 1984a, p. 122–129)

FURTHER CORRESPONDENCE ABOUT RAILROADS, MASS TRANSIT, AND BEEPERS

Chicago, Illinois
January 20, 1984

Dear Mr. Engelken:

This will reply to the November 21, 1983, article about the opening of the Baltimore subway.

Over the years, I have followed, with anticipation and excitement, the construction and opening of new rail rapid transit systems, as well as improvements on older ones. As a blind person and transit professional, I must express serious concern with regard to a relatively minor system specification which ironically has major implications for a particular segment of the transit riding public—the blind—as well as the ridership in general. The Mass Transportation Administration of Maryland (MTA) contends that beepers above rapid transit car doors will make the Baltimore system more accessible to blind passengers. It is significant that this is the only system in the United States with beepers that sound as rapid transit car doors open. No other rapid transit cars now being manufactured or delivered to U.S. properties have this feature. Even Dade County, Florida, which jointly ordered cars with Baltimore, does not have beepers on its cars.

Ironically the beepers, intended to assist the blind, may in the long run have the opposite effect. Blind persons who have not ridden rapid transit trains in other cities may develop the false notion that their safety in boarding subway trains in Baltimore is directly related to the beepers. They may rely on the beepers and may pay less attention to the sounds of doors opening and the footsteps of boarding and alighting passengers. The beepers might also distract them from hearing these sounds. If the train stops so that the end entrance door is nearest the blind passenger, he or she would have to choose between boarding through that door without the aid of the beeper, or running up to half a car length (about thirty-five feet) to a center entrance door with a beeper. Those who learn to rely on the beepers may have difficulty in boarding trains if beepers malfunction. Such blind passengers would have to board trains without beepers in other cities, such as nearby Washington, D.C. or Philadelphia. Blind persons accustomed to riding rapid transit systems in other cities may find the Baltimore beepers distracting and annoying. (That has been my reaction to audible traffic signals.)

More subtle, yet more serious is the reaction of the sighted community in the context of the misconception that public places and accommodations need to be specially modified for the blind. Since transit is most commonly used to travel to and from work, sighted riders may well discover that the beepers were installed on the misguided premise that blind passengers cannot board the train without them.

Blind persons are often asked how they will get to work or get around at the work place. Safety and higher insurance rates are often used as false reasons to deny employment to blind persons. The contention that public transit needs to be specially modified for the blind (as exemplified by the beepers) may, therefore, reinforce commonly held false notions which have historically kept the blind by and large underemployed or unemployed. I therefore feel strongly that the beepers should be removed.

I have been working for the Chicago Transit Authority (CTA) for over eight and a half years. I have been blind ever since I can remember. Except for the Baltimore system, which I intend to ride in early February, I have ridden every heavy rail rapid transit system in this country. I have also ridden transit in several Canadian and European cities, most recently London Transport and British Rail. Frankly, in all my rapid transit travels, it never crossed my mind that beepers were necessary to alert blind passengers that train doors have opened and to indicate their location in relation to where blind persons are standing on the platform. The door mechanism, whether air or electrically operated, as well as the footsteps of other passengers, provide adequate sound to serve that purpose very well. If these sounds are obscured by loud background noise—such as expressway traffic, construction equipment, low-flying planes, or oncoming trains—the blind person can use the cane to walk up to the edge of the platform then walk along side the train to the nearest open door. The cane also alerts the passenger as to whether a space is an opening between cars or a doorway. As such, the passenger can board safely and quickly. Blind passengers using dog guides also board trains safely and quickly.

I am a member of the National Federation of the Blind, the largest and most progressive organization of the blind, with more than 50,000 members nationwide. It has been our experience that blind people who have developed self-confidence and a positive attitude about themselves can travel competently anywhere they wish on all modes of public transportation. The Federation has, therefore, taken the position that special modifications for the blind (such as beepers) in public transportation and accommodations are unnecessary and promote negative attitudes toward blindness among the blind and the sighted. The philosophy of the National Federation of the Blind is that given proper training and opportunity, blind persons can lead active, normal lives and can compete on terms of equality with their sighted neighbors.

Cordially,

Steven Hastalis
(Jernigan, 1984b, pp. 128–131)

Chapter 5

DISCOURSE, DOMINATION AND RESISTANCE: NEW IMAGES FOR THE BLINDNESS SYSTEM

We are all familiar with images about blindness and other disabilities which appear in literature, advertisements, the mass media, and in the everyday speech and humor of ordinary citizens. However, little attention has been paid to the images about blindness created by professionals and to the power relationship reflected in the resulting discourse. In this chapter we will examine new images created by experts from 1936 to 1965 who referred to science for legitimacy in explaining blindness in the United States. We then discuss the harmful aspects of this image creating process in the efforts of rehabilitation workers and educators of blind people to establish for themselves an autonomous new profession. Finally, we analyze consumer resistance to these new definitions of blindness and the perception that some research and academic scholarship is self-serving for professionals and harmful to blind people.

Karl Mannheim (1936) developed a sociology of knowledge perspective in the tradition of Marx. He focused on the relationships between the intellectual point of view held and the social position occupied and found that new ideals and images became embedded in discourse, not from the random utterances of individuals, but from newly developed and established interest groups. Neither mankind in general nor isolated men and women create new traditions of thought; rather people participating with others in interest groups develop a similar style of thought as they continually respond to similar situations and issues (Mannheim, 1936). Sociologically and historically, Mannheim clarifies how the interests and purposes of certain social groups come to find expression in theories, doctrines, and intellectual movements. Astronomers continually create new concepts to explain the universe. Microbiologists continually create more adequate explanations of genetic transmission. Nutritionists and health educators create and disseminate new explanations of the relationship between nutrition and health. All call themselves professionals. Most are granted recognition for their specialized knowledge and accomplishments and all are relatively well paid for their efforts.

This process has also happened in the field of rehabilitation. It is different, however, because the objects being studied, manipulated, educated, rehabilitated or managed are other citizens. Those focusing on the ideology created by interest groups frequently have not taken sufficient account of power relationships. As we examine the history of discourse about blindness, we will find that the creation of new ideas about blindness has enabled workers and educators in the field of rehabilitation to claim exclusive domination over economic resources and employment opportunities. The recipients of these rehabilitation efforts have seldom had any alternatives for assistance. If not wealthy, they had only state agencies or privately funded "lighthouses" which operated in most major cities. The person seeking rehabilitation had no choice but to accept the definition of his or her situation provided by agency personnel. If the educator or rehabilitation worker had a narrow view of the employment potential for blind people, the result for an individual client was correspondingly restricted. Resistance, such as insistence on training for an occupation or profession not considered appropriate for a blind person, could result in a diagnosis that the client was not well adjusted, that he or she had not accepted his or her blindness. We can better understand the power relationships within the rehabilitation field by analyzing discourse about blindness and the resulting resistance of many blind people to recurring patterns of domination.

Michel Foucault (1974) examines the historic development of patterns of domination and how patterns of language facilitate domination. "It seems to me that the real political task in a society such as ours is to criticize the working of institutions which appear to be both neutral and independent; to criticize them in such a manner that the political violence which has always exercised itself obscurely through them will be unmasked" (p. 171). Power refers to the control some have over others. It may become manifest in prison walls, or, as is more usually the case, in the minutiae of social arrangements. In this case, I am not so much interested in the language and discourse as I am in the resulting practices and procedures and the consequences these have for individuals seeking autonomy and responsibility. Through his analysis of historical discourse, Foucault studied forms of domination including prisons, mental hospitals, clinics and scientific discourse about sexuality during the Victorian era up to the present. He reviewed the rise of medical language which gave increasing power to physicians, psychiatrists, and men, in general, over women. He wrote,

> The object, in short, is to define the regime of power-knowledge-pleasure that sustains the discourse on human sexuality in our part of the world. The central issue, then (at least in the first instance), is not to determine whether one says yes or no to sex, whether one formulates prohibitions or permissions, whether one asserts its importance or denies its effects, or whether one refines the words one uses to designate it; but to account for the fact that it is spoken about, to discover who does the speaking, the positions and viewpoints from which they speak, the institutions which prompt people to speak about it and which store and distribute the things that are said. (1978, p. 11)

If the word "blindness" were substituted for "sexuality" in the preceding quote, and "advantage" for "pleasure," we would have a good account of our objective in this chapter. Foucault's analysis parallels the recent history of discourse about blindness. Although a topic for later in this chapter, his analysis of architectural and institutional control arrangements could equally apply to workhouses, asylums and special institutions for controlling the behavior of blind inmates. For example, in his discussion of the "docile body," Foucault described the minute details of training that transformed the peasant into a soldier. Discipline also frequently requires enclosure—separating into homogenous groups those to be disciplined and regulated. "There was the great 'confinement' of vagabonds and paupers; there were other more discreet, but insidious and effective ones. There were the colleges, or secondary schools: the monastic model was gradually imposed; boarding appeared as the most perfect, if not the most frequent, educational régime" (1977, p. 141). Through architectural and other social arrangements, thought patterns of subordination and domination, and the new language used by most people and internalized by blind individuals, they became The Blind. Hence, another category was added to the array of groups being regulated, and each individual experienced this pervasive and subtle domination (Mizruchi, 1983). "These methods, which made possible the meticulous control of the operations of the body, which assured the constant subjection of its forces and imposed upon them a relation of docility-utility, might be called 'disciplines' " (Foucault, 1977, p. 137). The ideological thinking of "professionals" in recent decades has increasingly come into conflict with that of blind people themselves. Enlightenment through improved education has led to a transformation of social relationships between client and expert. Oppressive, arbitrary and frequently frustrating programs have been questioned. Empowerment begins to appear when subordinated individuals unit in their own organizations and begin to create alternative views about the nature of their own condition. Becoming independent, self-directed, responsible for oneself and actively trying to assist others in their search for autonomy does, on the face of it, appear laudable. However, Mannheim and Foucault would not be surprised to learn that challenges to old ideologies and positions of advantage have frequently met resistance.

As an observing participant, I was initially puzzled by the conflict and degree of hostility between consumer organizations of blind people and some of the organizations and professional groups claiming to educate and rehabilitate them. The growth of the organized blind—in terms of legislation, self-help, education of the public, and the efforts to develop the human potential of blind people—would appear to be consistent with the frequently stated goals of rehabilitation programs. However, many blind people are now questioning their value and, indeed, the very assumptions about blindness held by some members of those occupational groups who provide rehabilitation and educational services.

Scott observed in *The Making of Blind Men* (1969) that blindness is a learned social role. Attitudes about blindness are acquired in early childhood through daily interaction with other people and from organizations established to help blind people. Professional workers are often quite important because they enter the socialization process at the crucial moments when blind individuals seek employment or educational opportunities. Fortunately, there have been a number of important studies about the activity or work of individuals who claim blindness as a field requiring specialized training for professionals. Spector and Kitsuse (1977; 1987) analyzed the process of defining social problems and the activities that promote this process. For them, the definitional activity constitutes the social problem. Gusfield (1975; 1982; 1989) examined the struggle for organizational ownership of problems and the subsequent production of supportive scientific claims about them.

An assumption of this chapter is that the relative amount of visual stimulation available to people is not an "objective" condition. This assumption is shared by Scott and is consistently affirmed by the leadership of major organizations of blind people. Sociological interest focuses on how claims about conditions are created, documented, and extended. Largely ignored in research on this topic, however, are definitional activities that precede professional and related bureaucratic developments (Schneider, 1985).

When institutions and programs to serve blind people and other recipients of public assistance were first established in the United States, welfare, protection, and education were the most common goals proclaimed. The sense of mission of workers for the blind has arisen from definite understandings of the seriousness of blindness as a condition. These understandings "constitute vital sources for a sense of professional esteem, client respect, and the ability to maintain a legitimate occupational place. They constitute the source of belief that a knowledge base has been buttressed by the methods and expertise of scientific and technical professionals" (Gusfield, 1982, p. 44).

Several scholars locate the origins of public care for the blind in the Poor Laws of Elizabethan England (French, 1932; Katz, 1986; Koestler, 1976; Matson, 1990; tenBroek and Matson, 1959). Distinctions between indoor relief and outdoor dole were established at this time. The outdoor dole was aid provided to individuals and families in non-institutional settings. Indoor relief referred to asylums—residences or institutions intended to house the poor and infirm.

During the period 1830 through 1860 many asylums were established in the United States. "Removing deviants, including the poor and infirm, from society, placing them in an institution and providing a strict regimen was the best approach for solving social problems that were associated either with prisons, insane asylums, or almshouses" (Rothman, 1971, p. 191). Welfare was now the primary responsibility of the state; individual and religious group charity declined in importance.

Paralleling the widespread development of asylums, special purpose institutions were also developed to educate and otherwise care for individual categories of disabled people. Schools for the blind developed in almost every state during this period, and the Perkins School near Boston, Massachusetts, became a model for the education of blind children. Such schools did not replace the welfare asylums, but provided a special niche for educable children. These schools for the blind were influenced by those in Germany, France, and England. Johann Wilhelm Klein started one of the first programs oriented around education—not charity. His was a school, not an asylum. He started the Vienna Institute for the Education of the Blind in 1808, and by 1816 his program attracted so much attention that his school was elevated to a state institution receiving royal support (French, 1932, p. 103). "Certain categorical programs were set up at a state level in recognition of the fact that numbers of blind and deaf children or other specialized groups were too few in local areas to warrant proper facilities" (tenBroek, 1948, p. 45).

Whether in general asylums or specialized schools, many blind people were "cared for" in the general context of charity and welfare. Neither the discipline and poverty of almshouses nor specialized schools resulted in significant economic or social improvement of the lives of inmates (tenBroek and Matson, 1959). Still, programs proliferated and new agencies were created. Almost every major city developed a "lighthouse" supported by private philanthrophy. Funds available from state and federal sources grew steadily. Those in charge organized themselves as teachers (American Association of Instructors for the Blind) and, later, as comprehensive welfare workers (American Association of Workers for the Blind).

Commenting on the failure of the asylum movement, Rothman observes that the funders of the almshouses lacked special training. They also, frequently lacked formal education. "There was nothing very interesting, let alone exotic, about decrepit and unemployed men, and nothing that would confer a special status on those who managed them" (Rothman, 1971, p. 193). Educators of the blind argued that the unusual needs and condition of blind people required dedicated teachers with specialized skills for educating and otherwise helping blind people. Despite sympathy for blinded veterans of World War I and the authorization of federal funds for state programs, the understanding of blindness and the potential of blind people changed very little.

In 1932 the American Foundation for the Blind published *From Homer to Helen Keller,* a widely acclaimed social history of blindness written by Richard French, who for twenty-two years, until his retirement in 1946, had been director of the California State School for the Blind. A review of some of Dr. French's opinions about blind people sadly illustrates what were widely held ideas in the 1930s. Even worse, not a single article or comment appeared in *The Outlook,* the dominant journal for workers for the blind of that day, criticizing the ideas of this prestigious educator and administrator. For French, one hundred years experience in education of the blind had led to an accumulation of facts which were to be "conceded" by those who had given the subject much thought: Music is overestimated as a vocational area; the blind can do first class work only in a few handcrafts—basketry, weaving, knitting, broom-making, brush-making, and chair-caning; the blind cannot compete equally with the sighted in quantity or quality of items produced; crafts pursued by the blind are best done in workshops, supervised by government officials or officers of benevolent associations; apprenticeships and commercial education can help prepare blind persons for work; sales and shopkeeping are promising fields for those "sufficiently fortified in soul" to handle failures; among the "higher" callings, piano-tuning and, under favorable conditions, massaging are fields with the greatest possibility of success; teaching and other learned professions are, on the whole, only for those with superior talent; and, "To argue from individual success is not to show what the 'blind as a class' can do, and that therefore many notable examples of success, whatever their moral worth may be, cannot be taken as other than exceptional and therefore as practically valueless in the formulation of general guiding principles" (pp. 200–201).

Later in the same book French observes that a blind woman of normal intelligence and good health should have the right to marry and rear children. He states that there are some charming blind women and that a man able to support a wife and children may well choose to marry a blind woman. However, "[f]or two helpless blind persons to be mated as public charges and to bring children into the world, whether congenitally defective or not, is the height of folly: worse than that, it is a crime and one that ought to be made impossible by law and law-enforcement" (p. 230).

Enter Science

About the same time that French's book was published, presentations were made at meetings of educators and workers for the blind, and articles appeared in *Outlook for the Blind* reflecting new knowledge based on science and psychoanalysis. A review of conference proceedings and all issues of *Outlook for the Blind,* beginning with 1907 clearly shows that the 1930s was the decade when appeals to science entered the field of "work for the blind." Several of the ideas in this section also appear in my article "New Images for the Blindness System" which appears in the February, 1993, issue of the *Journal of Rehabilitation* (Volume 59,1). French hoped "that practice could be rationalized, that scientific method and a logical critique could successfully be applied" (pp. 250–251). Unfortunately, much of what all this faith in science brought was demeaning and debilitating.

In a 1931 article, "Psychological Problems of a Newly Blinded Adult," Dr. Holsopple, a clinical psychologist at New Jersey State Hospital, frequently drew analogies between the behavior of young children and that of newly blinded adults.

> As the child, tired from a long day's play, fails to recognize his desire for sleep, cries for attention and gets it only to burst into tears a moment later when he discovers attention is not so satisfying after all, so the adult newly blinded may reach for one satisfaction after another only to find disappointment with all attainment. (Holspopple 1931, p. 37)

Infantilizing was to become a frequent theme in describing the behavior of blind people. While citing Freud concerning the importance of sexuality to blind people, Holsopple recommended that competent psychological advice should be sought. It might be OK for the blind to have sex, but celibacy was preferable: "The satisfaction of desires other than sexual and the cultivation of these other satisfactions may lead to a happy substitution" (p. 36).

Psychologists, particularly Dr. Samuel Hayes, adapted existing intelligence, achievement, and vocational aptitude tests for use with blind students and the Perkins School for the Blind became the showcase for these "new psychological services" (Farrell, 1934). In addition to modifying the Binet-Simon and other tests for use with the blind, Hayes published more than twelve articles in *Outlook for the Blind*. The first, published in 1933, was "Problems in the Psychology of Blindness," in which he wanted to correct misconceptions about blindness and "to show the many interesting unsolved problems which await the patient application of reliable scientific methods for their proper solution" (p. 209). In his second article (1934), Hayes reviewed an array of empirical studies from experimental psychology which indicated that blind people, contrary to public opinion, were not superior in hearing, touch, taste, and smell. In one study, blind people were rotated on barrels to show that their sense of balance was not extraordinary.

The experimental psychology which Hayes reviewed for readers of *Outlook for the Blind* dealt with physiological and psychological reactions from thresholds of perception to thresholds of touch. Unfortunately, he did not deal with the socialization or even the characteristics of blind persons. In all that he wrote concerning these empirical studies he argued that blind people were ordinary. He thought he was using science to dispel myths about blindness, but his narrow focus only dispelled myths about physiological responses. However, unlike all of the other writers who brought scientific rhetoric to the discussion of blindness, he consistently did not contribute to stereotypes concerning the inherent limitations of blindness and their effects on the personalities of blind people.

In 1934 a sociologist from Carlton College, Northfield, Minnesota, observed blind students and deemed them both opinionated and stubborn. The students could not see both sides of a question; they were either right or wrong (Sidis, 1944). Her generalizations were based on observations remembered from her experiences as a teacher of blind high school students.

Dr. Berthold Lowenfeld, who was first a Director of Educational Research for the American Foundation for the Blind and later a successor to Dr. French as head of the California School for the Blind, named three basic ways in which blindness restricted the individual, and thus created a paradigm which dominated professional thinking for the next three decades. He repeated his three limitations in almost every article and public presentation that he gave from 1944 through 1952. As usual, no other writer challenged these new "insights" which were considered further evidence that blind people were different in basic ways from sighted individuals.

First, Lowenfeld claimed, since visual sensation cannot be adequately replaced, the blind person is limited "in the range and variety of his concepts . . . These limitations in the perceptual field cannot but result in a restriction of the range and variety of ideas and concepts in blind individuals" (1944, p. 32). Second, the blind person is limited in mobility, and "dependent upon the aid of others, thus afflicting his social relationships and attitudes in varying degrees" (p. 32). Third, because a blind person cannot experience the world visually, he has less control over his environment. Because he cannot learn and thus conform to appropriate social behavior through observing and imitating others, he will become isolated. "The isolating effect of this detachment restricts the blind individual in his control of the environment and results in increased feeling of insecurity and a state of higher nervous tension" (1947, p. 33).

Lowenfeld's three propositions about blindness were related to many other aspects or assumptions about blind people and he claimed that the "effects of blindness also tend to drive the blind individual into a world of unreality and fantasy where he may find compensation for his real or supposed failures" (p. 34). He also argued that sight is essential in order to carry on the ordinary activities of life (p. 31). Furthermore, he accepted the results of intelligence tests that there are fewer blind persons of average and superior intelligence and many more than the general population that are dull, border-line, and feeble-minded (p. 35). Concerning achievement, although blind children begin on a similar level, they fall increasingly behind with each year of education. However, Lowenfeld did not consider the quality or appropriateness of the education received by blind students as a possible explanation of their relatively poor performance on achievement/intelligence tests: "Besides blindness as such—which affects particularly the information component of the tests—heredity, poor environment, illness, emotional conflicts and late admission to school are some of the factors which contribute to the unfavorable distribution of IQ's and to the educational retardation" (1944, p. 35). Congenitally blind individuals, he thought, were worse off than the partially sighted or those totally blinded in later life.

Subdividing blindness led to the creation of new language and even occupational specializations. For example, some vision is better than no vision. To lose vision at age twelve is better than having lost it at age six. There are people with "partial," "high partial," and "shadow" vision. The greater value attributed to some residual vision is communicated to the blind person who calls himself or herself partially sighted rather than blind.

Lowenfeld was still discussing his "three limitations of blindness" as late as 1962. In a review of psychological studies of blindness, Kirtley (1975) mentions the same ideas. Santin and Simmons (1977), in "Problems in the Construction of Reality in Congenitally Blind Children," reflected and cited Lowenfeld's "limitations" of thirty years earlier. Since sight is our chief contact with the objective world, the input from the remaining senses is intermittent, elusive, sequential, and necessarily received in fragments (1977). The partially sighted can be treated by low vision specialists. When vision further declines, a new specialist takes over. Such distinctions have resulted in intense debates over the best approach to the education of blind people, and we will look at them in greater detail at the conclusion of this chapter.

Lowenfeld published more than one hundred books and articles about blindness. His perspective broadened somewhat in some later publications such as *The Changing Status of the Blind* (1975). In this book, he focused on factors associated with the integration of blind people into society and provided important historical material on the origins of self-help organizations. Unlike most writers in his field, he wrote favorably about the importance of consumer organizations such as the National

Federation of the Blind. Dr. Jacobus tenBroek, founder of the NFB, is one of the people to whom he dedicated this book.

In summary, Lowenfeld provided a series of ideas that defined blindness, particularly congenital blindness, as a condition which separates blind people from others in their access to "reality." Such people required assistance and could not adequately control their own environments. Also, almost any vision was better than no vision. Furthermore, the congenitally blind were worse off in any area he discussed than the adventitiously blind. Finally, as did other people, he repeated these ideas numerous times in the dominant professional journal of workers for the blind. As we have shown, workers for the blind who invoked science to help legitimate professional aspirations developed and spread images about blindness which were not only negative but which further divided blind people and ordinary people. Hence, appeals to science have led most to believe that the blind are stubborn, frustrated, out of touch with reality, disoriented, and necessarily dependent.

Historical Diversion Concerning Progress

More than two-hundred years ago, in *Emile* (1762), Rousseau's treatise on education, a different tone and attitude towards blindness was reflected.

> We are not masters of the use of all our senses equally. There is one of them—that is, touch—whose activity is never suspended during waking. It has been spread over the entire surface of our body as a continual guard to warn us of all that can do it damage. It is also the one of which, willy-nilly, we acquire the earliest experience due to this continual exercise and to which, consequently, we have less need to give a special culture. However, we observed that the blind have a surer and keener touch than we do; because, not being guided by sight, they are forced to learn to draw solely from the former sense the judgments which the latter furnishes us. Why, then are we not given practice at walking as the blind do in darkness, to know the bodies we may happen to come upon, to judge the objects which surround us—in a word, to do at night without light all that they do by day without eyes? As long as the sun shines, we have the advantage over them. In the dark they are in turn our guides. We are blind half of our lives, with the difference that the truly blind always know how to conduct themselves, while we dare not take a step in the heart of the night. We have lights, I will be told. What? Always machines? Who promises you that they will follow you everywhere in case of need? As for me, I prefer that Emile have eyes in the tips of his fingers than in a candlemaker's shop. (1979/1762, p. 133)

We also note Rousseau's concerns that machines might not always be available for one's needs. Those who promote "safety" for blind people at occasional places might take notice. In some areas it is easy to question the amount of progress made in the past two hundred years. Through professional imagery, claiming science for legitimacy and engineering and architectural efforts for promoting safety, we have developed ideas about blindness that have regressed from those portrayed in Rousseau's writings.

Professional Self-Understanding

Although workers for the blind had published a journal since 1907, they did not discuss their occupation as a profession at their annual meetings nor in their literature until 1939–1942 when several presentations were made and articles were published extolling the virtues of professionalization and standardization. In the twenties and thirties workers had been lauded as humane and involved in a "noble calling." Now claims were being made that this work was not only a profession but a specialized activity due to the peculiarity of the problems of blind people. Ph.D.s were now more common after the names of professionals, and quantifiable, positivistic research appeared frequently. When Wilensky (1964) observed that an occupation will not be granted professional status if its claims are based on common sense or easily codified procedures, he well may have been describing the field of workers for the blind.

Harry Best, a sociologist at the University of Kentucky, was one of the featured speakers at the 1939 annual meeting of the American Association of Workers for the Blind (A.A.W.B.) where he decried public misunderstanding of the profession:

> It is our solemn obligation to make the public understand that we are engaged, not in a formless, shapeless, disorganized, straggling enterprise, and one reeking with sentimentality, but one that can be and is being placed upon a foundation made of solid rock, and that can be carried on in an efficient, businesslike, dignified manner, and according to the fullest principles of commerce or industry or other pursuit known to man. The circumstance that we are engaged with the noblest of all human causes should not bar us from proving that we are likewise engaged in an undertaking that can meet the strictest standards of professional and scientific endeavor. (p. 203)

In 1941 Samuel Hayes referred to social work for the blind as a fast developing new profession. The "News and Views of the A.A.W.B." section in *Outlook for the Blind* reported in October, 1941, that home teaching was the first area in which workers needed to establish professional standards. Committees were working and resolutions were passed as early as 1939. The June, 1942, "News and Views of the A.A.W.B." reported that "progress was made in setting up standards for home teachers and preparing for certification of workers in this field" (*Outlook*, 1942).

Partly because of increased federal funding for vocational rehabilitation programs, Robert Irwin, nationally prominent as head of the American Foundation for the Blind, focused attention on the specialized nature of work for the blind. In "Why Rehabilitation of the Blind is a Function of the Special Agency for the Blind" (1943) he argued that "unusual special services" are necessary. Because of the severity of the handicaps of blind people, their rehabilitation is more difficult and calls for special knowledge. The best results come from agencies specializing in services to the blind:

> Because blindness affects all phases of an individual's life—even such simple matters as eating, dressing, reading one's personal mail, walking down the street alone—and also because the psychological effects of blindness are probably more severe than for any other type of physical handicap, vocational rehabilitation of the blind is as much a matter of social case work as it is of vocational training and placement. Therefore the rehabilitation of the blind is more appropriately a function of a social agency, such as the commission for the blind or the department of welfare, than of a department of education. (Irwin, 1943)

Objections to existing ideas and the work of other professionals are rare in the literature of workers for the blind. In fact, we found only two examples of articles explicitly written as critiques. Foulke (1972) did challenge previous ideas about the personalities of blind people as being "not very helpful." Mettler (1987) not only critiqued previous ideas, but also provided new and positive ways to view the adequacy of sensory information available to blind people. A lone voice, he argued that different modes of sensory perception need not result in significant social differences.

Consumer Resistance

The National Federation of the Blind was organized in 1940. Dr. Jacobus tenBroek and many others continually claimed that with proper education and enlightened public attitudes, blind people were as ordinary as anyone. In his 1948 Presidential Address to the Ninth Annual Convention, tenBroek expressed this philosophy as he argued for a bill of rights. Several articles by Dr. Kenneth Jernigan and many others calling for a reinterpretation of the significance and meaning of blindness appeared in the widely circulated consumer journal, the *Braille Monitor* (1982a; 1982b).

When domination occurs, even those on the bottom have some power, as has been demonstrated in mental institutions, P.O.W. camps, civil rights movements, prisons and many other settings. Resistance comes through informal sub-cultures or overt noncooperation. Agencies have power over those requiring rehabilitation services because they have resources needed by the client—assistance in job training, placement, educational services, and so forth (Adam, 1978). Only in the largest cities do blind people have alternatives for opportunity. Even then, the agencies and programs are usually similar. As we noted at the beginning of this chapter, domination is easier when clients internalize the definition of the situation created by professionals or others in positions of power.

The NFB leadership recognized that a group becomes empowered when it organizes itself around a new identity. Then the behavior of those who dominate can be changed when the group refuses to recognize their legitimacy and begins to question their policies, programs and philosophies. In our case, power is grounded in the self conceptions of those in subordinate positions (Fay, 1987). For this reason, agencies and many professionals have supported the equivalent of company unions. The American Council of the Blind is a consumer organization which in its publications never questions existing established programs or agencies. The opposite has been true of the NFB, which seeks to alter the self understanding of the membership through a positive philosophy repeatedly shared through seminars, support groups, local chapters, national conventions and a monthly journal. "We are changing what it means to be blind" and "we know who we are and we won't go back" are two of the most frequently heard themes.

In 1976 Dr. Hanan Selvin, a prominent sociologist, reflecting on his own experience of encountering blindness in late life, wrote that with proper training blindness may be viewed only "as a nuisance." Ideas about blindness, he noted, were a larger concern than the physical condition itself. Soon thereafter, Paul Schulz (1977) published what appeared to be a rebuttal entitled "Who Says Blindness is Just an Inconvenience?" Those who denied the severity of blindness were not mature. Sight is the best sense receptor and source of information and it has no equivalent. Many responses appeared in both consumer and professional journals (Cobb 1977; Jernigan 1982a; Olson 1977). Changing what it means to be blind became a major theme as the Federation worked to present "more positive" images of blindness.

Conclusion

We have shown that professional ideology began in early images of philanthropy and gradually called on "science" for legitimation, later represented most frequently by Lowenfeld's "three limitations" of blindness. This symbolism defined blindness as a severe condition which separated blind people from the reality experienced by others. Charitable acts were not enough: the blind needed highly specialized workers for their rehabilitation and education. At almost the same time those understandings of blindness were being diffused, arguments appeared for the "professionalization of the field." Professionalization included licensing and accreditation requirements, with the American Foundation for the Blind coordinating developments.

The new imagery about blindness and professionalization of the field, along with the publication outlets and professional networks, were each heavily influenced by the American Foundation for the Blind. Beginning in 1940, however, professionals encountered a well organized and rapidly growing consumer movement. The National Federation of the Blind argued for the equality, competitive employment, and full consumer participation in programs for blind people. With a more informed public understanding and proper education they could be both independent and as "normal" as others.

The conflict between providers of services and consumers mentioned at the beginning of this chapter is more than symbolic; it is resistance to domination. Critics of the "blindness system" argue that it is harmful to blind individuals, that it causes dependency, internalized negative self-images, and unnecessarily negative public images. Educators and rehabilitation workers have major interests to protect—agencies, endowments, programs, and increases in federal and state funding. Shepherding the growth of career opportunities is important in a narrowly defined work arena. Excluding blind individuals by judging them incapable of teaching mobility helps protect the opportunities for the existing pool of workers as well as those for prospective new employees being trained in the small group of university centers specializing in blindness rehabilitation.

In the fifties and sixties most rehabilitation counselors considered few occupations suitable for blind people. Because federal and state rehabilitation regulations in many states prohibited pay for graduate education, it was the exception when a blind person was encouraged to become a lawyer, schoolteacher, computer programmer, physician, or businessman or woman. Today, blind people are employed in all of these fields. Vocational rehabilitation counselors have expanded their horizons as a result of pressure from blind people themselves. Now there are countless examples of how negative self images have been offset by positive role models and strong support networks. The following letter by Ken Silberman (February, 1991) including introductory remarks by Barbara Pierce (1991b), the associate editor of the *Braille Monitor,* illustrates how autonomy and self determination have led to accomplishments which could not have been envisioned twenty years earlier.

THE PROOF OF THE PUDDING

From the associate Editor: One of the most satisfying aspects of watching the years roll by as a member of this movement is observing the growth and maturation in people who have joined the organization more recently. As a member of the Scholarship Committee in 1985, I was assigned the task of notifying Ken Silberman, an astronomy major at the University of Pennsylvania, that he was one of the year's winners. His file was impressive. In addition to his academic work in a field which I could not fathom, he indicated that he had been a member of a volunteer fire department and had done scuba diving.

We talked at length by telephone several times that spring, and I came to understand that Ken, like so many others, was doing some remarkable things, but he had no real self-confidence as a blind person. He could not use Braille. He did not travel effectively or confidently with a cane. His alternative techniques for completing his mathematical and scientific work were inefficient and cobbled-together. In short, I did not hold out much hope for his future despite his impressive academic record.

I am learning, however, that one should never underestimate the power of the Federation's impact on a person of character and determination. Ken looked around that summer at the first truly competent blind people he had ever seen and decided that he wanted what they had. He took himself off to a rehabilitation program in which he really could master Braille and the use of the white cane. He earned a master's degree from Cornell in aerospace engineering, and he began looking for a job. He found one in data base management at the Naval Ship Systems Engineering Station in Philadelphia. But he has continued to nose around for something that would lead more directly toward aerospace program management. Meanwhile, he began working as a Job Opportunities for the Blind volunteer in Pennsylvania, which helped him to hone his own skills in job-hunting. Now it is all paying off. Here is a letter which explains what has happened and puts it all in perspective:

September 18, 1990

Philadelphia, Pennsylvania

Dear President Maurer:

It has often been said that change is the only true constant. I guess this is so. At any rate, I'm not doing anything to disprove this philosophy. On 21 October, I shall be starting work at NASA's Goddard Space Flight Center in the Space Data and Computing Division.

My job will involve researching and interpreting data from the archives in response to the queries of Astronomers. The data from all American (and some foreign) space missions is stored in these archives. It's time to put some of my undergraduate training to work.

It's not exactly what I want, but it gets my foot in the door. I had hoped to get into the space program from the military side. Oh well, there's more than one way to skin a cat. I hope to move into management. (Based on my experience in government, this is an area where my talents are desperately needed.) I plan to do a superior job, to learn what opportunities are available or can be made, and to use some political finesse to make helpful allies. Who knows? With a lot of hard work and a little luck, I might get to fly. After all, when the space station becomes a reality, they're going to need a lot of disciplines, not just fliers. I know this is a lot of dreaming. But, if you don't shoot for a target, you won't ever hit it.

A lot has happened since my first NFB national convention in Louisville. I've gone from being a mess to being one of the best in 5 years. Back then, I didn't believe that a blind person could do very much. However, after being touched by the Federation and its leaders that summer, I could only conclude that Ken Silberman couldn't do very much. And I was not prepared to be content with that. There was only one thing to do—get off my backside and get to work. Well, this job is the result. Not bad, eh?

As I close this letter, I am struck by the fact that I could not have achieved any more if I had been sighted. Of course, it would have been much easier if I had not had to overcome the handicap of the professionals who did their best to set up road-blocks in front of me. But, with the help of the Federation, I have done it. The proof of the pudding is in the tasting. I've earned this job. I deserve it. And I've got it!

Sincerely yours,

Ken Silberman

Organizations of blind people continually combat harmful images about blindness which appear in all types of media. For example, the NFB picketed, telephoned, wrote letters and contacted advertisers of ABC to protest the image of blindness portrayed in the 1991 sit-com "Good and Evil." The sighted actor, George, played the role of a blind man who was foolish, clumsy, and in other ways inept because of his blindness. Although the network had anticipated a full season for this show, it was cancelled after six weeks. The portrayal of blindness was so degrading that protest came from many people in addition to the organized blind.

Publishers apparently do quite well selling books to the general public about the heroics of disabled individuals, and many non-disabled benefit, probably more than Jerry's Kids, from telethons. Money raised from evoking pity for disabled children provides good advertising for corporations and luxury conventions for television executives and many others involved in fund raising. The huckstering continues despite the complaints and also picketing by various groups protesting the harmful depictions of disability.

The following article by Barbara Pierce (1991c) illustrates the continuous effort of blind people to oppose harmful images about blindness.

WHAT'S IN AN ATTITUDE

From the Associate Editor: I have a friend who is accident-prone. She walks into door jambs, slips off steps, stumbles over tree roots, and crashes into coffee tables. I have another who loses things and spends hours every week hunting for objects that have vanished into thin air. My husband is absent-minded. He depends heavily on his calendar, but I have learned through the years that part of my job in our family is to remember things for us both. All of these people happen to be sighted, and all are inconvenienced to one degree or another and at one time or another by these annoying traits.

All of us know dozens of people, including ourselves, who have these inconvenient little characteristics. They shape our lives to some small degree and have some slight impact on our personalities, but they do not define our characters or determine who we are. Generally we human beings are more interested in learning whether others are bright, competent, trustworthy, amusing, compassionate or cut-throat, dangerous, selfish, intemperate, bigoted. This is so unless the individual under scrutiny is disabled. Then character traits, good or bad, slide out of focus, becoming nothing more than repercussions of the disability—blind people are always cheerful or surly or patient or whatever trait the disabled person is exhibiting at the moment. Instead people concentrate on the superficial details of existence, blowing them all out of proportion: How does that person using a wheelchair negotiate stairs? Do the children of blind people always put their toys away? Can he really pick up that coin with a prosthetic hand?

As blind people, we have learned to tolerate this obsession with the unimportant in the general public. It arises from ignorance and can be combatted by patient education. Each of us is engaged in the struggle for enlightenment every day. It is, therefore, both dismaying and frustrating to find that a blind woman has weighed into the battle for truth and perspective on the opposite side. To make matters worse, she is clearly talented, competent, and ambitious. Her name is Sally Hobart Alexander, and she has written a book for children from the point of view of her young daughter. It is called *Mom Can't See Me,* and it contains virtually all the stereotyped notions and attitudes about blindness that we fight to eliminate or put in their proper perspective; Braille is hard to learn and difficult to use. Blind people bump into things and depend on others to keep obstacles out of their way. They can no longer teach school or even know much about what goes on around them because they can't depend on vision. All this comes from a woman who (also according to the book) has a good marriage, is successfully raising two attractive, well-balanced children; travels independently; goes canoeing; and in general lives a perfectly full and normal life.

The whole thing is a tragedy. Of course, Mrs. Alexander has the right to her view of the world and of blindness, and she is free to write a book that reinforces the negative stereotypes of blindness and magnifies out of all proportion the inconveniences we face. It is not surprising that the Macmillan Publishing Company would choose to produce the book; after all, it appears to the ignorant to be a refreshingly realistic portrayal of the daily burden of blindness. Only the blind are damaged by it. Only our efforts to educate the public about our abilities and competence are undermined.

Galley proofs of this book were sent without comment to Lorraine Rovig of our national staff in August of 1990. Publishers usually do this when they are soliciting reviews. Macmillan obviously hoped that the National Federation of the Blind would provide a glowing review that it could use in promotional materials. Sandy Halverson of Missouri and I happened to be at the National Center when the manuscript arrived, and Miss Rovig read it to us for our reaction. She then wrote to Macmillan in an attempt to explain why the book would be damaging to blind people. Of course, Macmillan has never replied to the letter and has on the contrary arranged the usual promotional book-signing and public relations efforts. We did not expect anything else. Contracts had been signed, resources were committed to the project, and editors were riding the fashionable wave of disability texts for children.

In the end, my predominant reaction to this book is pained regret that a woman with so much going for her seems to believe that she is courageously breasting the tide of misfortune. If she does not believe this, then she knows how lucky she is and has chosen to make money by exploiting the public's misconceptions of blindness. In either case our work has been made more difficult. We must reach a little deeper and try a little harder to demonstrate to the world, blind and sighted alike, that blind people are not defined by a few inconveniences. We must demand that the world focus on our accomplishments, not complications. Here is the letter Lorraine Rovig wrote to Macmillan Publishing Company:

Baltimore, Maryland
August 21, 1990

Ms. B. Lyons
Macmillan Publishing Company
New York, New York

Dear Ms. Lyons:

Thank you most sincerely for sending a galley copy of *Mom Can't See Me* by Sally Hobart Alexander, photographs by George Ancona. Unfortunately, although it has much to recommend it, it does not meet our criteria for progressive books about blindness and blind people. We could not recommend it to parents, teachers, or children.

No doubt you will wonder why. I wish you could have been in the room when I read the copy of *Mom Can't See Me* to two blind women, one from Ohio, the other from Kansas City, Missouri. Both are totally blind professional women, wives, and mothers, who are active in sports and social engagements; and both women were appalled at some of the attitudes evidenced by the author.

For example, neither woman believes she collects a great many bruises because she can't see. Both women have perfected their ability to travel well with the long cane. Both know other women who use guide dogs in similarly successful fashion. In fact, both women regularly travel around the United States independently for speaking engagements and other activities.

One woman believes that none of her children when young successfully stole cookie dough without her knowledge; the other believes her eleven-year-old son has a similar lack of success in fooling Mom. I'd like to note that, since Mom Alexander is writing this book, it seems odd for her to say that she doesn't know that her daughter is stealing cookie dough. But I wonder how many readers will notice the illogic of the statement made by the child. We three women expect that the general attitude held by the public will lead most readers to swallow the proposition that blind mothers couldn't possibly know what their children are doing. The National Federation of the Blind has had to go to court in many cases to get children returned to blind mothers or parents because some neighbor called a social worker, and the social worker kidnapped the children based solely on this proposition.

Both women recoiled at the strong suggestion that Mom cannot teach elementary school after becoming blind. No, the copy does not directly state this. Yes, most readers will leap to this conclusion. As the director of the National Federation of the Blind's national program Job Opportunities for the Blind, I can put Mrs. Alexander or you in direct touch with totally blind elementary school teachers with full-time and part-time jobs. However, principals and other hiring personnel will find that this book confirms their prejudices. *Mom Can't See Me* will put one more brick in the wall that blind school teachers must break down before being seriously considered on the basis of credentials and personality, as are other candidates.

My audience and I were particularly distressed that this book states, "Braille is hard to learn." We know individuals (with average intelligence) who have learned Braille in as little as two weeks. We know many, many children and adults who learned Braille or are currently learning it. The average length of time to learn Braille well is six months. You likely learned print when you were in first grade. It probably took you six months to learn the print code well. (No more mistakes in knowing a "b" from a "d" or forgetting the sound of a "th" and so forth.) Mrs. Alexander's daughter says she knows because "I tried it." Does this mean she studied Braille for five minutes whenever she decided to play being blind? Did she sit down on a regular basis with a teacher? Did she study the physical skill as you and I studied the print code?

Her mother is obviously intelligent. Did she have a teacher who told her directly or by implication that learning Braille is hard? Did her mother practice feeling the dots as recommended, for at least fifteen minutes each day? Have you heard the one about the self-fulfilling prophecy? One of the major problems facing blind children and adults today is the attitude of many professional teachers in special education that Braille is hard to learn. Without Braille many blind individuals are illiterate and lack sufficient skill successfully to handle a competitive job in the modern world.

All three of us feel confident this book will continue to reinforce the prevalent attitude about the incompetence of blind adults. We find this especially regrettable since the author shows a great deal of skill in writing and could have written a book with a much more positive and more realistic tone.

I've enclosed two articles written by blind mothers that were printed in our national magazine. Upon request, I can give you the names and phone numbers of these two authors and the individuals to whom I read the text of the book by Mrs. Alexander. Other material is available.

As soon as print copies of Mrs. Alexander's books are available for sale, we would like to purchase one copy of each title for our Research Collection on Blindness. We wish to acquire one copy of any book by a legally blind author or about those who are legally blind.

Again, thank you most kindly for sending a review copy.

Sincerely,

Miss Lorraine Rovig
National Federation of the Blind

There is currently a debate over the adequacy of mainstreaming as an educational alternative for blind and visually impaired students. Special education teachers are often not adequately trained for instructing blind children and may also possess negative images about blindness and the potential of blind students (see Chapter 8). Either from their professional training or from attitudes which abound in pop-culture, these teachers have often acquired many of the attitudes described in this chapter. Awareness of the poor education that blind students usually receive through mainstreaming has caused some blind people to reassess the strengths of the former schools for the blind.

Asylums or schools for the blind were thought to be both helpful and humane in the nineteenth century. The progressive era and mainstreaming in education brought an increased variety of opportunities. Residential schools still exist in each state; however, they emphasize educational programs for blind and visually impaired children who frequently have multiple physical or mental disabilities.

The literature appearing in the *Braille Monitor* frequently includes the complaints of parents seeking quality education for their blind children in the public school system. They allege that teachers often lack the skills to teach Braille and other necessary skills adequately. Positive peer support networks are frequently not available. Most blind people have rejected the custodial aspects of traditional residential schools, and they are equally troubled by the results of mainstreaming. This dilemma is reflected in the failed resolution described by Kenneth Jernigan in the September–October, 1988, issue of the *Braille Monitor.*

A THOUGHT-PROVOKING RESOLUTION AND AN ISSUE WHICH IS NOT YET SETTLED

Resolutions are the policy-making vehicles of the National Federation of the Blind, and usually the process is quite clear-cut. A resolution will be presented, discussed, and then voted up or down; and although the matter may again be introduced at a later time, for the moment it is settled. Not so with Resolution 88-21, which was introduced at this year's NFB convention by Rami Rabby.

It was not so much a resolution as an indictment of the present system of education of blind children. It called attention to the fact that the term "least restrictive environment," which is mandated by Public Law 94-142, is being used to promote the very opposite situation; that many educators are confusing geographic proximity with true integration; and that sitting at the next desk to a sighted child does not necessarily prevent the blind child from having social isolation or an inadequate education. The resolution caused prolonged debate and serious soul searching.

Ultimately it was defeated—not only in the Resolutions Committee but also by roll call vote on the floor of the convention. But the size of the vote does not tell the story, for many of those who voted on the winning side had mixed feelings and cast their ballots with troubled hearts. Hardly a person could be found who would say that the present system is working. In fact, there was virtually unanimous agreement that it is bad, extremely bad. Then why did the resolution lose? Some felt that while it pointed out the problem, it did not offer a satisfactory solution. Others felt that such a new approach (yes, *new* not *old*) should not be adopted too precipitously—that it needed more study, more discussion, and more refinement. Still others felt that (regardless of the resolution's merit and even conceding its correctness) its provisions would have no chance of acceptance throughout the country at the present time and that it would only serve as a vehicle for our opponents to attack us.

Yet, with all of these reservations, everyone agreed that the resolution spotlights a problem which must be dealt with. Braille is deliberately being de-emphasized in the education of blind and visually impaired children; skills are not being taught; and concepts of the inferiority of the blind are being sanctified and institutionalized by the very schools which should be teaching the opposite. Whatever the final form of the policy and plan of action which we adopt, the problem demands attention and solution. Between now and the Denver convention next year all of us should think about it and be prepared to deal with it. Here is the resolution, not as Rami Rabby originally presented it to the Resolutions Committee but as it was revised and defeated on the convention floor:

WHEREAS, the Education of all Handicapped Children Act (Public Law 94-142) is funded on the principle that every handicapped child in the United States shall be provided a free and appropriate education in the "least restrictive environment;" and

WHEREAS, this principle has been generally interpreted to mean that, merely by placing a disabled child in a regular public school classroom alongside his/her nondisabled peers, the environment automatically becomes less restrictive; and

WHEREAS, this attachment to physical mainstreaming as the paramount objective in the education of blind children has led to the virtual demise of programs in which blind children are instructed and trained in groups; and

WHEREAS, the National Federation of the Blind has always believed that the quality of a blind child's education is determined not so much by *where* the child is taught but rather by *what* is taught and *how* intensively—that is, whether or not the child is trained to develop a positive attitude about blindness, a healthy self-image as a blind person, and a self-confident, independent, resourceful, and problem-solving approach to life, as well as the basic skills of blindness, such as the use of Braille and the ability to travel with a cane, and to view these alternative techniques as efficient tools for success in today's society; and

WHEREAS, after observing the Education of All Handicapped Children Act in action since the mid-1970s, the National Federation of the Blind has reached the conclusion that the principle and practice of physically mainstreaming blind children (no matter what) have, for the most part, failed; and

WHEREAS, this failure is conspicuously reflected in the large numbers of blind high school graduates who, throughout their educational careers, were *physically* integrated but *socially* outcast, who consequently become unassertive, passive, and psychologically ill prepared to interact as equals with their fellow graduates, and who are woefully lacking in those basic skills of blindness which would otherwise have enabled them to compete head-on with their sighted peers, both in college and in the work place; and

WHEREAS, as more and more blind children are born into, and grow up in, two income families, it is not in their best interest to have career-oriented mothers and fathers sacrifice their need for self-fulfillment through work and instead spend their most productive years bickering and arguing in endless parent/teacher conferences, administrative hearings, and court appearances, in an heroic effort— usually fruitless—to convince teachers and principals to treat their blind sons and daughters as normal children and to instruct them effectively in the alternative skills of blindness; and

WHEREAS, it is the view of the National Federation of the Blind that, if mainstreaming is ever to have the slightest chance of succeeding, it is at a minimum absolutely essential that blind children be fortified with positive attitudes toward themselves as blind people and with the basic skills of blindness, *before* they venture into the competitive arena of the regular public school; and

WHEREAS, we believe that the sharing of ideas and information, common experiences, effective responses to negative public attitudes and practical solutions to blindness-related problems; the development of a strong sense of normalcy and a positive self-image; and the cultivation—through, for example, team sports—of that competitiveness, team spirit, and strategic way of thinking which are so crucial to later success in the world of work can, almost by definition, only take place in group settings, with the involvement of sizable numbers of blind children; now, therefore:

BE IT RESOLVED by the National Federation of the Blind in convention assembled this eighth day of July, 1988, in the city of Chicago, Illinois, that this organization call upon Congress, school boards and principals, the teaching profession, and all parents of blind children to redirect their attention away from the physical location of a blind child's education and toward its intrinsic substance and results, and to recognize that, in terms of the preparation of blind children for life as blind adults, it is *group* instruction of blind children rather than *individual* instruction of each blind child within the potentially unfriendly and frustrating atmosphere of a public school which, in fact, constitutes the "least restrictive environment;" and

BE IT FURTHER RESOLVED that, without in any way endorsing the poor equality of the residential schools for the blind as we know them, the National Federation of the Blind work toward the establishment of a nationwide network of specialized educational centers for blind children, whose precise location and character may vary, depending on local circumstances and conditions—for example, public programs versus private initiatives; city-wide day centers versus residential or semi-residential facilities drawing students together from largely rural areas—but whose purposes would be to evaluate the readiness of blind children for mainstreamed education and, if necessary, to train them until such time as they may individually be prepared, in their attitudes and competencies of blindness, to move to a regular public school and to compete on an equal footing, both academically and socially, with their sighted peers, in their own neighborhoods; and

BE IT FURTHER RESOLVED that the National Federation of the Blind, both as a national body and through its state affiliates, continue and redouble its efforts to enhance the substantive quality of blind children's education under this new system, by pursuing the following strategies, among others;

A. Counseling the parents of blind children and advising them of the benefits of early attitudinal and skills training and of the significance of delivering that training in group settings.

B. Assisting and guiding the parents of blind children in the ongoing reinforcement of positive attitudes and effective skills, within the family.

C. Conducting educational programs and seminars for special education teachers-in-training.

D. Monitoring and pressing for the improvement of the quality of programs offered by the proposed educational centers for blind children, and of subsequent services in the public schools, and

E. Establishing our own educational centers for blind children, which would serve as national and international models in the field of special education. (1988b, pp. 462–465)

Chapter 6

CONSUMER RESISTANCE TO ACCREDITATION

"Social control refers to the means by which groups influence or direct individuals" (Walton, 1990, p. 318) and has sometimes been referred to as the politics of morality. People are socialized, taught, regulated or in other ways persuaded or required to act in a prescribed manner. Thus, social control is based upon group expectations and the means groups use to bring individuals into compliance. When governments license professionals and when regional or national organizations accredit local schools, they empower individuals who then rule over others.

Most people, anarchists excluded, agree that some social control is necessary to protect us from fraud, bad drivers, and misuse of public money and to set standards for government and educational performance. However, social control can also be studied when we consider the history of resistance efforts by subordinated groups. As Walton says, "Social control involves more than a unified set of expectations dictated from the top down. It also includes resistance and conflict" (p. 320). Resistance may be manifested by individuals, groups or social movements. Resistance to social control which has been judged unjust or arbitrary provides much of the diversity of social history. Out of rebellion or resistance emerges new patterns of social regulation.

Societies have frequently provided regulations to control blind people. In Elizabethan England we had the Poor Laws; in France prior to the Revolution, special schools; in the United States during the nineteenth century, asylums, workhouses, poor farms, and more special schools. Our present century has witnessed a proliferation of public and private agencies to educate, rehabilitate and otherwise take care of blind people and those disabled in other ways—often keeping them in their place and out of harm's way while simultaneously eliminating begging and other public nuisance activities that impose upon the lives of "normal" people. At the present time there are more than 800 agencies, public and private, which compete for public support to provide services to the blind and visually impaired. Unfortunately, they are sometimes regressive in their educational and rehabilitation procedures, wasteful of public resources because they are ineffective, or counter productive when, while trying to raise funds, they project images designed to evoke pity and thereby spread negative ideas about the people being served.

To control groups such as blind people, organizations are created to impose standards. People with power, usually those controlling the largest and best funded organizations in a given area, arrange procedures to bring wayward or backward organizations into line. It took more than twenty years of organizational effort to establish a national accrediting organization to regulate agencies serving the blind and visually impaired, mostly because some agencies and many individuals resisted in the name of self-determination, autonomy and responsibility. Blind people began to insist that they be included in making decisions about programs and arrangements affecting their lives. Their resistance is well illustrated by the nearly fifty years of conflict between the organized blind—the National Federation of the Blind and the many local and national agencies that have provided services. In this chapter we will examine the national effort for a standards and accreditation process over which many of the battles were waged.

As indicated by the number of articles in the *Braille Monitor* and related journals, no single conflict has attracted more energy and displayed more acrimony than the struggle between the National Federation of the Blind and the National Accreditation Council for Agencies Serving the Blind and Visually Impaired. In the three decades preceding the establishment of the National Accreditation Council (NAC) there were many developments in the field of working for the blind. However, once the new agency came into being, and despite its goals and early successes, it was continually opposed by the National Federation of the Blind and ignored or boycotted by many agencies and professionals working with blind people. Much of the material below comes from Frances Koestler's social history of blindness in America, *The Unseen Minority* (1976), a book commissioned and published by the American Foundation for the Blind.

Historical Background

Before World War II most education of the blind occurred either in special institutions or schools, or in the home setting by itinerant teachers. Shortly after World War II rehabilitation centers began establishing themselves in several parts of the United States. The number of blinded war veterans and the financial support from the Veterans Administration were one source of growth. These centers, sometimes developed in tandem with sheltered workshops, tried to help blind people adjust to their blindness and learn skills, and evaluated them for vocational training or educational purposes.

As early as 1932 there was concern about the degree or adequacy of the training of home teachers of the blind. These teachers were almost all women and the majority of them were blind. Since they often found themselves interacting with the rapidly expanding profession of social work which was developing its own standards for educational requirements, home teachers organized and appointed their own committee to develop minimum standards of practice (Koestler, 1976, p. 291). Further impetus toward standards for those who provided service to the blind came from the federal government in the 1939 amendments to the Social Security Act. All persons employed in federally funded welfare programs would have to participate in a merit system. "Since in many states the commission for the blind was part of the state welfare department, home teachers would have to meet the same civil service standards as those of the sighted civil service workers employed in other facets of welfare assistance" (p. 291). As Koestler noted, the question arose concerning whether or not blind people employed as home teachers would lose their jobs and possibly be replaced by supposedly more qualified, sighted teachers.

In 1938 the American Foundation for the Blind held a special conference to work out the philosophy and principles of home teaching. As a result, the American Association of Workers for the Blind appointed a board for certification of home teachers and the new standards for two levels or classes were adopted by the 1941 convention. Class 1 required two years of college training with courses in social work and education. In addition, Braille, typing, and proficiency in six handicraft skills were required. However, four years of experience could be substituted for the two years of college training. Class 2 required completion of the college course work of Class 1 and at least one year of post-graduate training in social work. By 1947, sixty Class 1 and three Class 2 certificates had been granted (Koestler, 1976, p. 292). Following World War II, in addition to the increase in professionalization among home teachers, came the development of private and public rehabilitation centers for citizens at large, and special ones for blinded war veterans. North Carolina, Florida and Arkansas took the lead in establishing these centers, and by the late 1940s there were also a large number of sheltered workshops and, in every state, some type of school or institution for blind children.

During the 1950s development was rapid because of increasing support from the federal government in areas such as the Veterans Administration, the Office of Vocational Rehabilitation, and the Hill-Burton Act which made funds available for constructing rehabilitation facilities independent of hospitals themselves. Private agencies serving the blind were growing in both number and size in almost every large American city. In 1956 the Federal Office of Vocational Rehabilitation, along with the American Foundation for the Blind, sponsored a conference in New Orleans to establish principles and standards for work with the blind. Organizers invited carefully selected workers in the field of blindness. As Koestler notes, many of these were the same individuals who had met at previous AFB sponsored conferences devoted to standards and accreditation. "Out of the work of the seventeen people who spent five days in sub committees and general sessions came a set of precepts that largely foreshadowed the standards later adopted by COMSTAC" (p. 297). COMSTAC was the Commission on Standards and Accreditation of Services for the Blind, the immediate predecessor of the National Accreditation Council.

COMSTAC

Reporting as chairman of a 1952 committee to explore standards, Roberta Townsend stated to the 1953 AAWB convention that a lack of unanimity of thought and of standards had resulted in "many sporadic programs" and frequent duplication of services. Following her report, the AAWB adopted a resolution "asking that 'a manual of useful criteria and standards for the guidance of agencies' be devised and that it be done by the American Foundation for the Blind" (Koestler, p. 340). In the same year the organization issued another blunt report criticizing agencies which provided almost no services but which sought funds from the public ostensibly to help the blind. It noted that more than 600 agencies were making approaches to the public for support with sometimes counterproductive results. Eventually, the growing concern for standards led to the accreditation of agencies in compliance with agreed upon criteria.

The Veterans Administration, in accord with a 1954 amendment, made many additional funds available for various rehabilitation services. According to Koestler, Robert Barnett, then President of the American Foundation for the Blind, recognized that a structured process involving standards and a method of implementing them would be necessary to achieve the maximum benefits for blind people from the increasing proliferation of agencies and funds available for rehabilitative services. Following this lead, the President of the AFB Board in 1961 said, "It is not our intention that the American Foundation for the Blind will itself conduct a policing program but rather that it will arrange to expedite a service program of evaluation and accreditation which would find its authority in a democratic representation of all legitimate interests in this field" (p. 342). As we will subsequently demonstrate, the conflict that swirled around this accreditation effort resulted, in part, from confusion about the meaning of "democratic representation of all legitimate interests in this field." It later became a basic contention of the leadership of the only national organization of blind people existing at the time that not only were blind people not represented, but that the entire process leading to the National Accreditation Council was tightly managed by a small group of professionals and orchestrated by the American Foundation for the Blind.

In 1962 an ad hoc committee of the American Foundation for the Blind recommended that an autonomous commission be appointed to develop standards and regulations and to create a permanent accrediting body. "Thus was born the independent organization known as COMSTAC: the Commission on Standards and Accreditation of Services for the Blind" (Koestler, p. 342). The American Foundation for the Blind agreed to partially finance the commission's work while allowing it autonomy. For four years the AFB provided $300,000 and the activity of many of its staff members while an additional $138,000 was obtained from three private foundations and the Vocational Rehabilitation Administration. Although Koestler does not tell us how the twenty-two members of the Commission were selected, she claims they represented both major professional groups interested in work for the blind and some blind people themselves. The executive director of COMSTAC, Alexander F. Handel, and eight other staff members were released from their normal activities at the AFB to run the Commission. Many additional committees, with support services provided by the AFB staff, were formed to focus on different areas related to standards and accreditation. They were given guidelines, we presume, by the COMSTAC staff to make sure that they did not engage in blue sky speculations or "unduly lax criteria." According to Koestler, "Standards [were to] be formulated so as to set a level of acceptable performance below which no agency should fall, while simultaneously constituting a challenge to the better agencies to continue striving for improvement" (p. 343).

The resulting committee reports were reviewed at a conference attended by more than four hundred people in 1965 and combined and revised in "The COMSTAC Report: Standards for Strength in Services." This report recommended that an organization be established to carry out the accreditation process, and thus the National Council of Agencies Serving The Blind And Visually Handicapped was established in 1967 with Arthur Brandon, the former chair of the Commission, as its first president and Handel its new executive director. The founders of NAC projected a ten year plan during which time the organization would be supported with fees paid by the agencies seeking accreditation. To underwrite the program during the developmental phase the American Foundation for the Blind and the Vocational Rehabilitation Administration assumed the greatest burdens. By 1972 the NAC had accredited forty-seven agencies with approximately that many more involved in some stage of the process (Koestler, p. 340). Even by 1972 it was apparent that self sufficiency would not be attained by the NAC and that it would require an additional period of subsidizing. Koestler says that the enthusiasm was not unanimous and cites the two reasons for resistance on the part of some groups: Professional standards might threaten the positions held by some blind people who might not measure up to new requirements in public and private agencies, and the accreditation process might ignore workers' concerns about minimum wage, collective bargaining and other labor practice issues (p. 344). Consumer literature of the time, as we will see, reflects also that there was concern that a small group of self-designated professional staff people had their own agenda—to manage and control the field of blindness. Consumer groups particularly argued that they had been under-represented and even ignored in the COMSTAC process. However, before examining their position, we will review some of the early enthusiasm reported by the officers of the NAC as well as by some agencies who experienced accreditation.

The first accreditations were granted in 1968 and were lauded in the first annual report of the NAC. Its president, Dr. Brandon, commented, "The ferment continues. Out of it will come rising numbers of accrediting agencies giving even better service to the blind and visually handicapped. And even as the numbers grow, the ferment spreads." The first three accredited agencies were proud of their accomplishment and began immediately using the seal of approval on their stationary and in other places affording public recognition. "Announcement of accreditation brought well deserved public recognition" (NAC Annual Report, 1968). In this same first year a 342 page study guide was published by the NAC. The check list and rating scales intended to guide self-study covered eleven aspects of agency activity: function and structure, financial accounting and service reporting, personnel administration and volunteer service, physical facilities, public relations and fund raising, library services, orientation and mobility services, rehabilitation centers, sheltered workshops (in multi-service agencies), social services, and vocational services.

Writing in the journal, *Education of the Visually Handicapped,* V. R. Carter commented on the agency he administered in Arkansas: "I wanted the school I administered to get in at the ground floor and be recognized nation wide as a school with a quality program" (1980, p. 75). He indicated that the NAC's accreditation was the high point of his more than thirty year career at the Arkansas School for the Blind, and he argued that accreditation helped his school measure up to standards that reflected broad professional opinions rather than those of the local staff. A 1974 editorial by Donald Walker in the same journal reinforced the source of direction for the accreditation process. He explained in "Accreditation or Evaluation?" that the setting of program goals was not the responsibility of the professional staff (p. 125). He was even more explicit in a 1975 editorial: "Thus, as professionals, we are responsible and accountable to society or its representatives for designing and implementing a program which meets the needs of the population we serve. The selection of the goals for which we are to be accountable is primarily the responsibility of those in whose authority we operate the program" (p. 63).

The professional literature, as reflected in the two major journals of that time, did not criticize COMSTAC or the NAC. Instead, articles extolled the virtues of accreditation: The strongest agencies would be further challenged and the weakest improved; through the self study process staff members would be exposed to national perspectives and agencies would no longer be isolated; physical improvements would be featured in fund-raising appeals based on the need to be nationally accredited. Goals and standards for the seal of approval came from professionals—national leaders of the field—who were sensitive to the perspective of the wider community which provided the funding for services to the blind or visually impaired, and the NAC was the only source of this seal of approval.

The View from the Other Side

During the period discussed in this chapter, the National Federation of the Blind, founded in 1940, was the only broadbased organization of blind people and, hence, the only group from whom were heard murmurs of discontent. The *Braille Monitor,* for three years called *The Blind American,* focused on the harm caused by "custodialism"—any practice which diminished the independent living capabilities of blind people. While a fairly small group of carefully selected leaders in the profession were developing the process and agenda for COMSTAC, *The Blind American* was publishing articles about agencies and practices which, it alleged, provided either exploitive or unequal treatment to clients receiving rehabilitation. In May 1963 the journal described the firing of forty blind people from the Berkeley workshop of California Industries for the Blind. They were "laid off" because of their demands for better pay and their efforts to organize a labor union (Matson, 1963, pp. 3–4). In September, 1964, an article entitled "Struggle Against Odds" described the efforts of NFB members in New Mexico to obtain an orientation center for their state. "The fact that the voice of the blind was heard for the first time by the 26th state legislature galvanized agency personnel to protect their present program and prevent any future organized activity" (Gomez, 1964, p. 5).

During the years immediately preceding the creation of COMSTAC, as suggested by the articles in *The Blind American* and the *Braille Monitor,* members of the National Federation of the Blind and of other organizations such as the Blinded Veterans Association were working to improve the economic and social conditions faced by blind people. As indicated above, there were requests for new rehabilitation centers, union recognition of employees of sheltered workshops, demands for better pay for blind workers in these workshops, and the initiation of many types of legislation in many state governments and at the national level. Prominent national political leaders such as Senators Robert Kennedy, Vance Hartke of Indiana and Frank Moss of Utah spoke at the NFB National Convention in 1965 and praised the Federation's efforts on behalf of blind people. Clearly, the National Federation of the Blind was a growing force in the struggle for equal opportunities for blind people. As its journal suggested, the Federation frequently worked with private and state agencies in mutual efforts to secure improved legislation and new programs. However, there appears to have been almost no relationship between the rapidly growing organized movements of the blind and the relatively small leadership group which had been shepherding the effort to professionalize the field of "work for the blind" and which, in the period between 1960–1965, had been working to develop a national accreditation procedure.

COMSTAC was first mentioned by the *Braille Monitor* in July 1965 in an article entitled "Agency Conference on Standards Set." The article observed that the Commission, from the outset, reflected the views of the American Foundation for the Blind and its associated agencies. "Organizations of the blind themselves, such as the National Federation of the Blind, have been conspicuously absent from the roster of groups and individuals asked to formulate supposedly objective 'standards' to be applied to all organizations in the field" (tenBroek, 1965a, p. 29).

Many articles soon appeared claiming that the American Foundation for the Blind and a related social network of professionals were attempting to dominate and control all agencies as well as individual blind people. This idea is at the heart of a 1965 speech by Kenneth Jernigan, who was then Director of the Iowa Commission for the Blind. Jernigan observed that agency personnel not only reflected commonly held misconceptions about blindness but in additional ways contributed to the difficulties confronting blind people.

> Let me now say something about agencies and organizations doing work with the blind. Employees and administrators of such agencies are members of the public, too, and are conditioned by the same forces that affect other people in the total population. Some of them (in fact, many) are enlightened individuals who thoroughly understand the problems to be met and who work with vigor and imagination to erase the stereotypes and propagate a new way of thought concerning blindness and its problems; but some of them (unfortunately, far too many) have all the misconceptions and erroneous ideas which characterize the public at large. Regrettably there are still people who go into work with the blind because they cannot be dominant in their homes or social or business lives, and they feel (whether they realize it or not) that at least they can dominate and patronize the blind. This urge often expresses itself in charitable works and dedicated sincerity, but this does not mitigate its unhealthy nature or make it any less misguided or inappropriate. (p. 82)

Professor Jacobus tenBroek, founder and first president of the NFB, reflected the growing self-confidence of the organized blind movement in his banquet address to its 25th convention.

> The career of our movement has not been a tranquil one. It has grown to maturity the hard way. The external pressures have been unremitting. It has

been counseled by well-wishers that all would be well—and it has learned to resist. It has been attacked by agencies and administrators—and learned to fight back. It has been scolded by guardians and caretakers—and learned to talk back. It has cut its eye teeth on legal and political struggle, sharpened its wits through countless debates, broadened its mind and deepened its voice by incessant contest. Most important of all, it has never stopped moving, never stopped battling, never stopped marching towards its goals of security, equality, and opportunity for all the Nation's blind. (1965b, p. 86)

In his review of the previous decade tenBroek observed, "All of a sudden, in the furious fifties, the National Federation of the Blind was very much noticed. Our organizations became the objects of intense attention—if rarely of affection—on the part of the agencies, administrators, and their satellite groups which had dominated the field" (p. 89).

When the National Federation of the Blind was founded in 1940, its purpose was to empower blind people to take care of themselves rather than to be cared for. For the members it was important to make the distinction that the organization was the National Federation **of** the Blind, not the National Federation **for** the Blind. From its earliest days it sought equal treatment for blind people in society. Its members and leaders would almost certainly have opposed the National Accreditation Council in earlier decades. However, because the establishment of COMSTAC and the National Accreditation Council occurred in the 1960s, the decade of the Equality Revolution, the reaction of National Federation of the Blind members was probably more intense than it would have been at an earlier time (Gans, 1973). Almost every minority and gender group in the United States was demanding equal treatment. The convergence of the interests of these different movements brought political responses leading to the civil rights legislation of that decade. Self-determination and full participation were "in the air." Leaders in the blindness field could not have picked a less propitious time to launch a new program and organization which did not call for the full participation of blind people dedicated to their self-determination. President tenBroek was a nationally recognized scholar in the field of welfare rights, who joined in a number of social movements of his day.

In 1966 many articles in the *Monitor* evaluated the work of COMSTAC. In January an article analyzing some features of the COMSTAC report on vocational services acknowledged that it relied on the existing practices of both private and government agencies, and concluded that the status quo was not being challenged. "Lip service is given to self-determination and progressive concepts, but the new language and psychiatric jargon cannot hide the paternalism that dominates this statement on vocational services to the blind" (tenBroek and Matson, 1966a, p. 10). The *Monitor's* coverage of the developments of COMSTAC activities moved to a climax in the February 1966 issue, which contained three articles by anonymous agency personnel. Apparently, they thought their careers might suffer as a result of their candid remarks (tenBroek and Matson, 1966c, p. 1).

In the first article concerning COMSTAC's report on agency functions and structure, the author cited the idealistic introductory material but emphasized that high principles do not lead to meaningful standards. While advisory boards reflect the makeup of a community, no mention is made of including blind people on advisory boards. This is presumably non-accidental, but based on an underlying assumption that well-meaning citizens and professionals "in the field" best know what blind people need. "For no matter how thoroughly you organize any controlling or advisory body, of what use is this organization if there is no communication or advice from the people who know most intimately the problems, the needs, the aspirations of the blind—those who live with the problems?" (Anonymous A, p. 4).

In the second, another author observed that the standards for physical facilities were meaningless because they could not be met by all types of existing facilities.

> The attitude of the committee is the standard belief that the blind are physically helpless. Token references are made to "respect for their potentials for productive participation in society;" but this is conditioned a short time later by the standard calling for a special crosswalk or stop light for "those blind able to travel independently" on a crowded street near the facility. (Anonymous B, p. 28)

COMSTAC standards would institutionalize arrangements, such as special street crossings, which many blind people had already come to reject as dependency creating.

The writer of the third article commented that the COMSTAC Report on Mobility Instruction was actually regressive, because far more positive approaches already existed.

> The introduction states: "When an individual loses sight, he loses, among other things, the ability to move safely from one place to another." The positive qualities of this statement are startling only by their absence. One wonders how conducive to making progress in travel programs this approach

can be. Aside from its unfortunate connotations, this statement isn't literally true. A blind person does not lose ability to move safely. That is still present — all he needs is to develop alternative techniques to procure the information he formerly obtained by visual means. (Anonymous C, p. 52)

Throughout 1966 the *Monitor* continued to review each Commission report. In an article entitled "COMSTAC—The Clients' Big Brother," the editorial staff further examined the report on vocational services and found that although it condemned traditional sheltered workshops,

> The Committee proposes a regimen of vocational services which not only retains the sheltered shop for employment and training purposes, but which is tailored to fit blind persons who are to be "treated," "trained" and "placed" by properly qualified "professionals". . . . [The] reader looks in vain for some recognition of the concept that blind people are persons who should enjoy the same opportunities as their sighted fellows rather than being objects to be "treated," "trained" and "placed." (tenBroek and Matson, 1966b, p. 45)

Clearly, many of the leaders of the nationally based, democratically elected, and largest organization of blind people were critical of the philosophy and motives of COMSTAC. The Commission was criticized for being regressive, for ignoring significant consumer participation, and for attempting to institutionalize practices which perpetuated dependency. To many blind people, as well as to several agency directors, the small group of professionals with similar and overlapping institutional affiliations was trying to dominate the field of rehabilitation through an organization which was straddled with negative and regressive assumptions about blindness.

The gulf between the organized blind movement and the professionals in charge of COMSTAC is perhaps best illustrated in a February 14, 1966, letter from the President of the National Federation of the Blind to Arthur L. Brandon.

> Your letter, I'm afraid, conveys the impression that you do not fully appreciate the cleavage between the blind and the professionals, so called, who have drawn up the COMSTAC standards. This is not mere trivial difference about formulation or desirability of this standard or that standard. Our position is far more fundamental. Indeed, for a parallel you should look to the Negroes and their Civil Rights Revolution. They will no longer be satisfied to have the whites exclude them and prepare standards of conduct for them. So with us. Our right to participate in the preparation of plans for our own lives and our own future — or if you will, in the formulation of standards for our institutions and services — cannot any longer be casually spurned as if it were an argument about the formulation of a standard or the punctuation of a sentence. That

right is not in any sense complied with by a form request to any of us to submit our views, which the professionals then may or may not pay attention to in their work on our lives. (tenBroek, 1966b, p. 26)

The other *Monitor* articles in 1966 criticized the lack of democratic proceedings in developing the COMSTAC standards—only professionals were involved in the important Commission membership and its study committees, while the elected representatives of the organized blind were ignored. Furthermore, some argued that a small, elite group of self-designated professionals was attempting to accredit firmly established facilities with outdated programs and philosophies that promoted dependence rather than independence for blind people. Finally, they warned that moving toward a national accreditation organization that could grant a seal of approval to agencies would strengthen the ability of a small network of professionals to dominate programs intended to serve blind people. The battle lines were more tightly drawn when the National Accreditation Council was formally established with the leaders of COMSTAC becoming its leaders as well, with most of the underwriting budget being supplied by the American Foundation for the Blind. These officers declined President tenBroek's offer to join the discussion by formally responding to articles appearing in the *Monitor*. Most publications of the main professional organizations—the American Association of Workers for the Blind and the American Foundation for the Blind— simply ignored the National Federation of the Blind. The conflict has continued more than 25 years with the largest organization of consumers demanding the reform of the NAC or the establishment of a new basis of accreditation.

Koestler's opinion was that opposition to COMSTAC and the NAC came from blind workers whose positions were threatened by professional standards. She noted that some groups objected to work conditions, labor practices, and low wages being paid in sheltered workshops, many of which were or would be accredited by the NAC. "The principal vehicle for opposition on these and similar grounds was the National Federation of the Blind, whose militant and outspoken president, Kenneth Jernigan, conducted a vehement crusade, first against COMSTAC and then against NAC" (1976, p. 344). We add, for historical accuracy, that President tenBroek and others were pointing out the principles which COMSTAC and the NAC violated as early as 1965–1966. However, to focus criticism on the national leadership of the NFB overlooks the almost endless array of resolutions appearing in almost every state convention, in almost every succeeding year, which criticized the NAC. This was usually done by citing alleged abuses and illegal practices which were frequently described in articles about NAC approved agencies. From reviewing the record, we have no doubt that the rank and file membership supported the democratically elected state and national leadership of the National Federation of the Blind.

In a 1991 convention address Jernigan made clear that the NFB's quarrel with the NAC was not a result of the concept of accreditation nor of efforts for improved services to blind people. "Many," he said, "felt that the AFB and federal rehabilitation officials (unwittingly aided by people of prestige in the broader community) would impose a system of rigid controls which would stifle initiative, foster domination, and take the emphasis off of real service and place it on bureaucracy, red tape and professional jargon" (1991c, p. 18). In the same speech Jernigan explained his perception of NAC and the way it operated.

> Federationists who attended the 1966 Louisville convention will remember that a report on COMSTAC and NAC was given at that time. I had been officially asked to serve on the NAC board. The offer was, of course, tokenism of the most blatant sort; and the question was whether to accept, leaving the Federation open to the charge of approving NAC actions, or to reject, exposing us to the charge of non-cooperation and leaving us with no means of observing and getting information. Federationists will remember that it was decided that I should accept the invitation. Thus, I have been a member of the NAC board since its inception. In the spring of 1970 I was elected to another three-year term. There are more than thirty NAC board members, of whom I am one.
>
> While expressing my minority views, I have tried to be personally congenial and friendly with the NAC board members. Nevertheless, tokenism remains tokenism. The other members of the board not only seem unconcerned with but unaware of the non-representative character of NAC. It is as if General Motors, Chrysler, Ford, and American Motors should set up a council and put six or seven officials from each of their companies on its board and then ask the UAW to contribute a single representative. What would the unions do in such a situation? What would racial minorities do if their representative organizations were offered such tokenism—in the establishment and promulgation of standards affecting their lives? I think we know what they would do. They would take both political and court action, and they would instigate mass demonstrations. Perhaps the blind should take a leaf from the same book. We cannot and should not exhibit endless patience. We cannot and should not forever tolerate the intolerable. I continue to sit on the NAC board, but I often wonder why. It does not discuss the real problems which face the blind today or the methods of solving those problems. In fact, NAC itself may well be more a part of the problem than the solution. I repeat that tokenism by any other

name is still tokenism. In May of 1969, for instance, I received a document from NAC entitled "Statement of Understanding Among National Accreditation Council, National Industries for the Blind and the General Council of Workshops for the Blind." This document was sent to all NAC board members with the request that they vote to approve or disapprove it. It contained six points, of which one and five are particularly pertinent. They are as follows: "1. by June 30, 1970, all NIB affiliated shops shall have either: a. applied to NAC for accreditation and submitted a self-study guide (or) b. applied to the General Council for a Certificate of Affiliation with NIB and submitted a self-study guide. 5. Certificates of Affiliation with NIB entitle shops to membership in the General Council and to access through NIB to: a. Government business allocated by NIB, b. Commercial business allocated by NIB, c. Consulting services of NIB, d. Any and all other benefits of NIB affiliation." In other words if a workshop for the blind wished any contracts from the federal government, it had better get into line and "volunteer" for accreditation by NAC. No pressure, of course, merely a system of "voluntary accreditation!" As you might expect, I voted no on the NIB agreement. Along with my ballot, I sent the following comments: "I do not approve this statement because I do not believe government contracts and other benefits to workshops should be conditioned upon their accreditation by NAC. Rather, receipt of government contracts and other benefits should depend upon the quality of performance of the workshop in question. Does the shop pay at least a minimum wage? Do its workers have the rights associated with collective bargaining? What sort of image of blindness does it present to the public?" (p. 21–22)

Over the next twenty years an average of seven articles per year appeared exposing alleged and documented short-comings of NAC accredited agencies. Up until 1990, the annual NAC board meetings were consistently picketed by 200 to 300 blind people who traveled to them from all over the United States. At the same time, others picketed the NAC accredited agencies in nearby metropolitan areas. In almost every state, federation members continually tried, often with success, to persuade agencies to disassociate from the NAC. The conflict has become a struggle with no middle ground. Meanwhile, the effort to criticize and discredit the NAC has been almost entirely ignored in the professional journals.

The Present Situation

However, in the past two years, due to a declining base of economic support and a failure to accredit even a small portion of agencies and programs serving the blind and visually impaired, the National Accreditation Council is in crisis and by only a slight margin failed to vote for its own dissolution. The January 1991 issue of the *Braille Monitor* listed

26 agencies, including dates of first accreditation and withdrawal (Jernigan, 1991a, pp. 40–41). In the same issue are listed 89 agencies which the National Accreditation Council claims as accredited through July 1990. Only ten of the fifty state agencies claimed NAC accreditation in 1990. In its early years, the NAC made a concentrated effort to accredit them, but from 1972 to 1977 this became a divisive issue in the National Council of Agencies Serving the Blind. Based upon telephone interviews with three current state directors, the issue of NAC accreditation has not appeared for serious discussion in the last decade.

According to Pinder (1991) in a recent survey of "knowledgeable leaders," probably members of the National Federation of the Blind, respondents were asked to identify "the ten worst vocational rehabilitation agencies in the country." Those surveyed did not know why the question was being asked, but "[i]n every single case, eight or nine of the NAC accredited agencies appeared on the list" (p. 25). It is probable that one could poll a group of leaders from the other major consumer organization, the American Council for the Blind, and elicit more favorable comments. Its publication, *The Braille Forum,* has never published an article critical of the NAC or any of its agencies. There are 71 schools for the blind listed in the most recent directory of services published by the American Foundation for the Blind, of which 26 are NAC accredited. Thirty-three of the 80 workshops listed by the National Industries for the Blind are NAC accredited (pp. 25–26). Even though the National Industries for the Blind agreed to pay for costs from 1986–1990, "only two workshops agreed to accept NAC accreditation while three dropped it" (p. 26). In sixteen states there are no NAC accredited agencies, while 33 agencies are concentrated in only four: Arizona, Florida, New York, and Pennsylvania. Fifteen additional states have only one NAC accredited agency each. Finally, thirty-one of the fifty states have a total of only 15 NAC accredited agencies.

In September 1991 in documents submitted to the Division of Accreditation and Institutional Eligibility staff of the Office of Post-Secondary Education of the U.S. Department of Education, the NAC reported a proposed budget for July 1, 1991, through June 31, 1992, of $216,065. This is considerably less than the budget reported by the NAC in its first annual report in 1968. NAC's peak year was 1986 when it listed 104 accredited agencies. As of December 1991 it had no more than 95 accredited agencies. Since the 1990 annual report of the National Accreditation Council for the Blind, the New Jersey Commission for the Blind, the

Iowa Braille and Sight Saving School, and the Southwest Lighthouse of Lubbock, Texas, have ended their relationship with the NAC (J. Gashel, personal communication, September 5, 1991).

On February 21, 1991, the National Industries for the Blind officially announced that its funding of the NAC would cease in June, 1991 and the American Foundation for the Blind made the same decision shortly thereafter. On April 7, the NAC's board met and made an effort to reduce costs and streamline its operation, but the motion was defeated by a 10-4 vote. Then a motion was proposed "that the board of directors recommend to the membership . . . that NAC dissolve no later than May 31, 1991. . . . " This motion carried by a 12-2 vote (Megivern, 1991; Jernigan, 1991b). However, the board of directors learned that it could not dissolve the corporation because dissolution required a vote of the membership. Thus, a meeting was called for May 5, 1991, in New York City and Joseph Champagne, chairman of the board, presided. There were approximately ten voting members present and, with the proxies, the result was 53 for continuing and 48 for dissolving the National Accreditation Council (Megivern, 1991). At the executive committee meeting which followed Champagne and Vice-president Evelyn Ullman resigned their positions.

In her coverage of these events in the *AER Report,* the official newsletter sent to members of the Association for the Education and Rehabilitation of the Blind and Visually Impaired, Megivern mentions the NAC's financial difficulties and its failure to establish further linkages with agencies. Her review provides no interpretation or background information about the intense resistance efforts of the National Federation of the Blind and other state and private agencies to thwart the National Accreditation Council's leadership. She only reports that business goes on as usual. As noted above, the professional literature has continually ignored the opposition to the established accreditation process. In summary, according to its own annual reports, the NAC currently accredits fewer than 100 of the more than 500 agencies originally envisioned. Both consumer and professional organizations agree on the need for quality services and a workable accreditation procedure, but an approach which focuses on the outcome of rehabilitation efforts and which includes full participation of representatives of organizations of the blind and visually impaired is necessary before this need can be met.

On May 25, 1991, Dennis Thurman, Superintendent of the Iowa Braille and Sight Saving School announced that he had received approval from the appropriate public authorities of Iowa to discontinue NAC accreditation. In addition, he described a possible alternative approach.

> Outcome accreditation is a new concept. It does not examine standards. It bases its accreditation on whether or not you make valid plans for students, analyze the students' success, and then use that information to change your instructional program. We are very interested in that concept of accreditation. We are very interested in getting away from "You need this, this, this" to a system that says, "Your students learned this, and you can change to provide this." We think that it's a better way to approach education." (Pierce, 1991a, p. 501)

I am including the article "COMSTAC's Children" (tenBroek, 1966a) because it illustrates as early as 1966, the National Federation of the Blind's perception of what it judged to be the absence of Democratic procedures in the process that led to the National Accreditation Council.

COMSTAC'S CHILDREN—
THE INSTRUMENTS OF ACCREDITATION

COMSTAC described itself as an autonomous body of 22 persons. It emphasized that it had over 100 professional leaders on its 12 standards writing committees. It claimed that over 1,000 persons contributed to the development of standards. That is almost enough to make one think in terms of the pure democracy of the New England Town Meeting. But look at what has really happened. The A.F.B. literally begot COMSTAC. It handpicked this supposedly autonomous group. Through its consultants it provided the expert advice on problems of blindness. It paid most of the money—$255,000 of $401,680. The field of work with the blind and the blind themselves were put neatly into the position of having to hear the good news and to accept it. Development and growth of standards, instead of working up the pyramid from a wide base, were imposed from on top. Subtract a point from democracy's score.

Now comes the final act in a grab for control as neatly masked as one could hope to find. Theoretically, having developed its standards COMSTAC was to fade out of the picture, and a separate organization was to be established which would implement the accrediting system.

A COMSTAC Newsletter of May, 1965 headlined "Independent Accrediting Agency to be Established." It went on to say, "A far-reaching decision was recently made by the Commission to create a *new* and *independent* agency to administer an on-going, voluntary system of accreditation of local and state agencies for the blind on a national basis.

At its last meeting, held April 22–24, the Commission voted to accept the recommendation of the Long Range Planning Committee that the permanent agency should be organized *separate* from any *existing agency or organization for the blind.*" [Emphasis added]. The December, 1965 COMSTAC Newsletter tries to continue this impossible notion. It states: "The Commission endorsed the plan of establishing a separate, independent accrediting organization on or before January 1967. . . .

Tentatively it is proposed that the new organization will be governed by a House of Delegates made up of representatives of member agencies." Here is another promise of democracy in action; a promise apparently made to be broken.

Then, under date of March 15, 1966, came the document containing the proposed Constitution and By Laws for the "National Accreditation Council for Agencies Serving the Blind and Visually handicapped." It would indeed be difficult to produce a document which at once sounds so democratic and at the same time creates so authoritarian a system.

Again, as with COMSTAC, it would appear that this "Council" is to rest on a very wide basis of acceptance and participation. Article III of the Constitution starts to open the door to as wide a membership as possible—practically any agency or organization, whether it be involved in work with the blind or not, may be eligible to be a member of the Council. That sounds good, but Article III further states "Decisions on eligibility for, continuance of, and termination of membership in the Council are to be determined by the Board of Directors according to the By Laws." And now add this factor—the first Board of Directors which will be in control for the first two years of the Council's life will be appointed by COMSTAC. He who begets can easily control. Subtract another point from democracy.

Why in the world can not the organized blind and the agencies interested in joining the Council be asked to send representatives to a constitutional and organizational meeting? There is nothing unworkable in such a procedure; that would be the democratic process. A striking characteristic of this Councils' constitution, and one which parallels the same characteristics in the work of COMSTAC, is that the end products—the standards, the accrediting power, the Constitution and By Laws—are not growing out of the work of the people but are being imposed from above. The pretense at democracy is only that—a degrading sham. Are the organized blind and the agencies and workers in the field so childlike that they must have their organization formed for them and controlled by self-imposed experts?

Let us examine the By-Laws of this new "Council" and see further how nicely truth and democracy may be subverted. There are to be three classes of members in the Council. Accredited members—who will be voting members—are agencies and organizations providing services for blind persons. Organizations of the blind would not be eligible to be voting members of the Council. Provisional members are agencies which have applied for accreditation but which do not quite qualify. Provisional membership is a status which may not exceed three years. One supposes that at the end of three years the provisional member who has not come up to the mark will be cast into outer darkness. Affiliate membership is the third class, and it covers a multitude of things. These members could be from any agency or group or organization "concerned" with services for the blind or "such related organizations as the Board of Directors shall determine." There is another sort of anomalous category of membership called sponsors. These could be "individuals, corporations, foundations, organizations or associations" who can be elected on an annual basis by the Board of Directors. The provisional member, the affiliate member and the sponsor while non-voting—have privileges of the floor at annual meetings.

That the Council is to operate on the basis of seeming representative democracy is evidenced by Article III of the By Laws which list the bodies that shall carry out the functions of the Council. These bodies are; House of Delegates, Board of Directors, Executive Committee, Nominating Committee, Commission on Accreditation, Commission on Standards, Standing Committee, Ad Hoc and Special Committees.

The House of Delegates consists of two delegates from each accredited agency—"One non-staff person and one professional staff person." Also in the House of Delegates will be the Board of Directors, one non-voting delegate from each provisional member, each affiliate member and each sponsor.

The main function of the House of Delegates appears to be to elect the Board of Directors, the officers and the members-at-large of the Executive Committee. And, having done that, it will have abdicated anything resembling legislative power or responsibility. That it is to hear and approve what comes from above is made clear in Section 2.A.1 of Article III of the By-Laws which says the House of Delegates shall "Serve as an advisory and consultative body to the Board of Directors on questions of standards and policies referred to it by the Board." It may "Initiate recommendations to the Board of Directors for standards and policies." The power to advise, consult with and recommend is indeed a mighty power—a mighty small power.

Obviously the real power of the Council will rest with the officers of the Council, the Board of Directors and the Executive Committee. Examine the structure of these bodies and observe how they are so tied together that there is no system of checks and balances, and that complete control is going to be retained by the parent organization that establishes them. These bodies at first are not even going to be popularly elected.

If we set up an organizational chart based on the By-Laws the following picture emerges. There shall be five officers of the Council—a president, two vice-presidents, a secretary and a treasurer. The first officers will be appointed by COMSTAC. There shall be a Board of Directors consisting of the five officers of the Council plus eighteen to twenty four additional members. The first Board shall be appointed by COMSTAC. There shall be an Executive Committee consisting of the five officers, three directors-at-large, the chairmen of the commissions on standards and accreditation, and the immediate past president of the council. The first Executive Committee shall be appointed by the Board of Directors which, of course, already would have been appointed by COMSTAC. The President shall appoint the nine member Commission on Accreditation—the chairman of which must be from the Board of Directors. The President shall also appoint a six member Commission on Standards, the chairman of which must be from the Board of Directors.

The controlling power of the Council will have been appointed for two years by COMSTAC. COMSTAC begot the Board of Directors—two-thirds of whom will serve for at least two years. COMSTAC begot the first officers—who are automatically members of the Board of Directors— three of the five officers will serve for at least two years. The Board of Directors, begot by COMSTAC, in turn begets the

Executive Committee, which automatically has the five officers already begot by COMSTAC. The President, in his turn, having been begot by COMSTAC, begets the Commission on Accreditation and the Commission on Standards—the chairmen of which have to be members of the Board of Directors—which was begot by COMSTAC in the first place.

An interesting omission in regard to elections—there is no provision for nominations from the floor. All nominations for the Board of Directors, Executive Committee, and officers will come from a nominating committee.

Does it not seem strange that they will have had no representation—no chance to express their views? The blind will be most affected by these developments. The sad truth of the matter stands forth in naked accusation in the writing of the standards and in the formulation of the accrediting system, the organized blind have been excluded; their voices have been ignored.

Think now of the peculiar situation which is being created through the establishment by COMSTAC of this so-called Council. On the face of it all seems democratic and in the traditional American Way. The Council shall consist of a wide range of members. The members shall send representatives to a House of Delegates. The House of Delegates, although it has no real legislative power, will elect the administrative bodies to conduct the business of the Council. There is to be an elected Board of Directors, a set of elected officers, an elected Executive Committee. There shall be two commissions—one on accreditation and one on standards. The Accreditation Commission shall have a judicial function. There are, on the face of it, some checks and balances and some separation of powers. In reality the elected bodies and the commissions are so closely intertwined and overlapped that direction and control of all affairs will be in the hands of very few—far removed from any supervision by an elected representative body. And more to the point, and more blatantly undemocratic, is the fact that the Council is going to have to operate for its first two years under appointed authority and with no means for participation by the membership.

Regardless of the reason COMSTAC may have—the blind and the agencies that serve them are witnessing a disgusting grab for power that may well cripple any forward looking movement to improve the situation of the blind in this country. (pp. 15–19)

For more than twenty years articles have appeared in the *Braille Monitor* exposing discrepancies between NAC's seal of approval and agency performance. One of the most common complaints has been about the exploitation of blind workers—that they are paid less than the minimum wage, that they are paid less for comparable work than sighted employees, and that they are seldom employed in management positions. These complaints concerning a NAC accredited agency are illustrated in the following article by Charles Brown which appeared in the May–June 1988 *Braille Monitor*.

THE RICHMOND WORKSHOP

Some time ago Ed Peay, President of our Richmond Chapter, wrote to George Kogar, Deputy commissioner of the Department for the Visually Handicapped, and asked him thirty questions about the Virginia Industries for the Blind facility located in Richmond. Mr. Kogar answered Ed's questions in a letter Ed received at the end of November of 1987. We think many of you will be interested in Mr. Kogar's responses to the questions.

According to Mr. Kogar's letter, there are thirty-three blind workers and two trainees employed in the workshop. All of the blind workers are employed in direct labor. All of the supervisors and management personnel are sighted. Only fifteen of the thirty-five blind workers receive the federal minimum wage. All of the sighted production workers, of course must receive at least the federal minimum wage.

Mr. Kogar also states that "The average annual earnings of a production worker is $6,676.80 per year." Remember that this figure includes the relatively higher earnings of the sighted production workers who must be paid the minimum wage. Mr. Kogar goes on to say that "The average for non-production workers is $11,264.26." Again, remember that all of these folks are sighted. One sometimes wonders if the Virginia Department for the Visually Handicapped is operating a sheltered shop for the sighted rather than a sheltered shop for the blind.

There is the additional matter of layoffs. Mr. Kogar informs us that "the industry has laid off blind employees on two occasions over the past three years. . . . No sighted employees were laid off during this time period. . . . The average duration of a layoff for a blind employee would be about eight weeks of intermittent work."

In his cover letter Mr. Kogar, to his credit, concedes, "The Industry has not been managed well for a long period of time. It will be a slow process to correct all of the problems of the past." In this regard the workshop director was let go last year.

Long-time Federationists know that we have been pointing out problems in the workshop for years. Officials have promised us that things would get better. They have not.

During all of this time, anyone who picks up a VDVH brochure or sees the agency letterhead finds proudly displayed the NAC symbol. This symbol proclaims that the agency, and its workshop, was fully accredited. Everything was deemed to be okay. We the blind are just troublemakers. NAC, everyone was told, would assure that blind people would receive "quality services." Without NAC who knows what might happen to the VDVH programs? Well, for one thing, people might have paid attention to the problems that exist in the Richmond workshop a lot sooner if VDVH had not chosen to hide behind the fictitious NAC shield. But all that is water over the dam. Yet, what are we, the blind of Virginia, to believe when in spite of everything VDVH Commissioner McCann tells us that he is "wedded to NAC?" (pp. 228–230)

Members of the National Federation of the Blind continually and almost at every opportunity educate, lobby, and otherwise try to influence agencies to sever their association with the National Accreditation Council. Sometimes it is through political influence when state agencies are concerned. Frequently, private agencies, such as Recording for the Blind, Inc., and The National Braille Association, disaffiliate for other reasons. It is in their interests to avoid the controversy which is frequently associated with the NAC. By withdrawing, they get only low level pressure from the relatively small group of professionals still enthusiastic about this particular form of accreditation. The good will which comes from blind people seeking a new accreditation process and enhanced opportunities for economic support appears to be a factor in the decision. This is illustrated by the following article which appeared in 1987.

THE NATIONAL BRAILLE ASSOCIATION
CUTS ITS TIES WITH NAC

As everybody knows, the last couple of years have been a bad time for NAC (the National Accreditation Council for Agencies Serving the

Blind and Visually Handicapped). The North Carolina School for the Blind, the Michigan State School for the Blind, Kansas State Services for the Blind, Rhode Island State Services for the Blind, and others decided they had enough and withdrew. There is an old saying to the effect that nothing wins like success. The reverse of that coin is that nothing loses like failure—and NAC certainly offers graphic testimony to the truth of it all.

One of the latest to leave NAC's sinking ship is NBA (the National Braille Association). Established in 1945, the NBA is described in the 1984 edition of the American Foundation for the Blind's *Directory of Agencies Serving the Blind in the U.S.* as follows: "Brings together those interested in production and distribution of Braille, large type and tape recorded materials for the visually impaired. NBA Braille Book Bank provides thermoform copies of hand transcribed texts to college students and professional persons; NBA Braille Technical Tables Bank has a collection of over 300 tables which supplement many of the texts; through NBA Reader-Transcriber Registry blind people can obtain vocational daily living material—at below cost; through Braille Transcription Assignment Service; requests of college students for Brailled textbooks are filled. Publications to aid transcribers include: *Manual for Large Type Transcribing and Tape Recording Manual, 3rd Ed.* available from LC/DBPH; *Teacher's Manual and Tape Recording Lessons,* from NBA national office; *Guidelines for Administration of Groups Producing Reading Materials for the Visually Handicapped,* from LC/DBPH; *Handbook for Braille Music Transcribers,* from LC/DBPH; and NBA *Bulletin,* issued four times a year to membership, available in print, Braille, or tape."

This is how the National Braille Association is described by the American Foundation for the Blind. Put briefly, it is the nationwide organization of transcribers. It has both prestige and stability. It has been one of NAC's sponsors from the very beginning. Therefore, its withdrawal must be particularly troubling to NAC. When we learned of the NBA defection, our reporter called NBA officials for comment. First we contacted Angela Coffaro, the staff member in charge of NBA's headquarters in Rochester, New York. Ms. Coffaro seemed uneasy at discussing the matter but said she thought that financial considerations were only partially involved in the NBA board's decision to withdraw sponsorship of NAC. She seemed to feel that the critical point for the NBA board was that NBA and NAC simply "had no basis for a continuing relationship." She did not explain why, if this is true, there was "the basis for a continuing relationship" from the late 1960s until now. Ms. Coffaro said that, even if it had wanted to, NBA could not be an accredited member of NAC but only a sponsor. She said that there was, therefore, no purpose to be served by NBA's remaining as a NAC sponsor. Ms. Coffaro said that the decision to withdraw was entirely the NBA's and that NAC simply responded with "regrets." Ms. Coffaro offered the thought that she believed other NAC sponsors were reaching the same conclusion that NBA had reached. She seemed reluctant to discuss the matter at all, expressed the opinion that it might be just as well if no publicity were given to the situation, and finally referred the *Monitor* reporter to Ms. Betty Crolick of Fort Collins, Colorado, NBA's President.

If possible, Ms. Crolick seemed even more uneasy about discussing the NAC withdrawal than Ms. Coffaro had. She confirmed the fact that the National Braille Association had definitely withdrawn its NAC sponsorship, and she said that the reason was not the amount of the annual dues for sponsoring members. She said the dues were only $50 per year and were really not a factor in the decision.

Ms. Crolick expressed her belief that NBA was one of the original NAC sponsors, dating back at least to 1970 when she originally joined the NBA board of directors. She said she could not comment on the exact reasons for NBA's withdrawal from NAC, but she went on to say that NBA and NAC seemed to have very little in common and that none of the NAC standards would seem to be relevant to any of NBA's activities. Beyond that, Ms. Crolick would only say that it was "just no longer appropriate for NBA to continue membership in NAC." She expressed the hope that NBA's withdrawal from NAC "would not become the center of publicity." She explained that this was why she would have to decline to give further reasons for the NBA–NAC separation.

The restrained statements of Ms. Coffaro and Ms. Crolick speak with more force than loud denunciations. The facts speak for themselves. From the very beginning of NAC (for at least almost twenty years) the National Braille Association has lent its name and prestige to NAC. All of that has now come to an end. Why? Surely NBA and NAC have as much in common now as they did twenty years ago, and as both NBA representatives emphasized, the nominal amount of dues for a sponsoring member was not a factor.

The plain truth is that NAC (if it ever had a constructive part to play in the field of work with the blind) has such a part no longer. The greatest service it could possibly render would be quietly to dissolve and go out of existence. If it does not soon voluntarily do so, the job will almost certainly be done for it—and with a great deal more pain to NAC than if it just quietly went away. (Jernigan, p. 326–328)

Chapter 7

AGENCIES AND PROFESSIONS:
THE CONSUMER RESPONSE

In 1969 Robert Scott published the first sociological monograph on the socialization of blind people. He noted that blindness is a learned social role which is acquired through the ordinary processes of social learning (p. 14). Scott described three contexts in which individuals learn behavior patterns and attitudes associated with blindness. The first is early childhood socialization, the second is immediate social interaction with sighted individuals, and the third is the organizations established to help blind people. By 1968, Scott had counted more than eight hundred such organizations in the United States. "In highly industrialized societies such as our own, the responsibility for the management, control, and rehabilitation of blind people is rested primarily in specialized organizations, most of which are large, complex, bureaucratic structures" (p. 18).

Scott considered it impossible to exaggerate the importance of these organizations in the lives of blind people. In fact, he argued that the phenomenon of blindness has been transformed by these agencies and programs. The very existence of special segregated institutions in the community defines the condition as unusual and requiring special intervention. According to Freidson (1965),

> It should be clear that the management of deviance is quite capable of organizing deviant behavior in that labeling or implying a label for it stimulates the community to organize its response to the individual, to a degree segregating him by those special responses and encouraging him to behave—to accept the role of the blind man, the village idiot, or the cripple. (p. 71)

The special institutions established to take care of blind people in this country include schools for the blind, sheltered workshops, special program centers (usually called associations for the blind or "lighthouses"), and residential rehabilitation centers. In addition, there are national organizations, such as the American Foundation for the Blind, and federal and state vocational rehabilitation programs. These special places are locally well known because of their fund raising appeals and public relations efforts. They may be housed on large campus-like sites, such as the Lion's World Center in Little Rock, Arkansas, or in a single building or office space shared with other public organizations such as family service or state welfare programs. The larger may employ two hundred or more people and own property which, in some cases, could conservatively be valued at more than $200,000,000, such as nearly two blocks of Manhattan owned by the American Foundation for the Blind in New York City. On the other hand, an agency like the St. Louis Society for the Blind has only seven or eight employees housed in a small office building. With endowments, continuous fundraising, bequests, and monies from the United Way, government and other business contracts, such agencies have fairly stable cash flows and gradually increasing annual budgets.

Institutions for the blind represent economic assets as well as ongoing economic resources, both for communities where they operate and for the individuals who manage and are employed by them. Almost all have boards of directors or public advisory boards, and except in unusual conflict situations, they are in large part controlled by the staff. Rapid turnover is not a characteristic of upper level management in this narrowly focused work arena because the mobility opportunities are limited for those working in blindness rehabilitation and its program management.

In addition to the establishment of organizations created to help blind people, in the past fifty years there has been a continuing effort to professionalize those occupied in blindness rehabilitation and education. There now are several large national organizations of workers and administrators, such as the Association For the Education and Rehabilitation of the Blind and Visually Impaired (A.E.R.), the National Council of State Agencies for the Blind (N.C.S.A.B.), and the Council of State Administrators of Vocational Rehabilitation (C.S.A.V.R.). There are also organizations for principals of schools for the blind, sheltered workshop directors and private agency groups. These organizations reflect national networks supported by newsletters, journals, university training centers and frequent state, regional, national and international conferences. These occupational groups usually define themselves as professionals and claim to apply to the many individual cases they attempt to rehabilitate or educate a body of knowledge that they profess to be especially privy to. As Scott noted, "The legitimacy of this profession is in large part based upon its practitioners' claims to specialized knowledge and expertise concerning problems of blindness" (p. 18). They create and disseminate "knowledge" about the condition of their clients, and their activity is another major source of ideas about blindness and about which behaviors are appropriate for properly adjusted, "cooperative" clients. In almost all cases, these workers are employed in the agencies and organizations mentioned above. Regardless of the degree of professional autonomy claimed, those who work in blindness rehabilitation conduct their activities in bureaucracies—formally organized work settings.

In this chapter we examine some of the consequences of rehabilitation services when they become subordinated to organizational or professional interests, and we focus on the conflict which emerges when clients and client organizations challenge the legitimacy of professional claims and activities. Of course, all of the agencies and professional associations were originally created to aid blind people and over the decades have helped bring blind people together. They also have been frequently successful in educating blind men and women, many of whom began to reflect on their own situations and to question the adequacy or appropriateness of services offered to them. By 1950, it was already evident to many leaders of the organized blind movement that blind people and agents of rehabilitation shared few common interests. "The idea that there is a unity of concern or interest between those at the top who bestow their benevolence and those at the bottom who receive it is open to doubt" (Gusfield, 1989, p. 436).

Sheltered Workshops

Sheltered workshops originated when religiously motivated people sought to "take care of" the disabled and blind. It was better for them to be sheltered than "on the streets." Of course, their concerns were for the spiritual well-being of their charges—employment and rehabilitation were usually secondary.

In France as early as the 13th century, organizations were developed under royal patronage to care for blinded crusaders, not dissimilar in motive to the programs instituted in the United States following World Wars I and II (Vaughan and Vaughan, 1993). In 18th century France a special school was established which contributed to the tradition leading to present day sheltered workshops, as part of the modernization of French society preceding and contributing to the Revolution. King Louis the XVI was so impressed by such efforts that he subsequently provided funds for the school, which he visited on December 26, 1786.

> At a special school for blind children — the first of its kind in the world — run by Valentin Haüy, the younger brother of the great mineralogist, the King witnessed the miracles of enlightenment, benevolence and skill. Twenty pupils, all of them blind since either birth or infancy, read out loud from books specially printed in raised relief-print, identified places and features on maps, sang and played musical instruments in his honor. The older children were also able to set type, spin yarn and knit hose. Especially impressive was an eleven-year-old boy, Le Sueur, who had been the first of Haüy's pupils, discovered pathetically begging for himself and his seven brothers and sisters, and who now was the prodigy of the class, almost a teacher in his own right. A few months earlier the Academy of Music had the first of a number of benefit concerts for this "Philanthropic School" and the King was moved and impressed enough to endow it with special funds and scholarships. A similar institution run by the Abbeé L'Epée cared for deaf-mutes and had invented the first lip-reading system, which enabled his charges to lead a normal and evidently happy life. (Schama, 1989, pp. 188–189)

In the 19th century, educators of blind people failed to anticipate societal resistance to the employment of the newly educated blind. Graduates began to return to their schools. School reports reflected inquiries from former students seeking help for employment. (Best, 1934). Thus educators of blind people became disillusioned and abandoned goals of equality and integration because they could not place their graduates in competitive employment. It was soon generally agreed that the solution to the problem could only be found in the creation of subsidized shelters where the blind might ply the simple skills learned in school, without harm from competition — or contamination — from the sighted (tenBroek and Matson, 1959).

One result was the sheltered workshop movement, which educated blind people for specific work tasks. Some of the material for this chapter also appears in my article "The Social Basis of Conflict between Blind People and Agents of Rehabilitation" (1991). In *Hope Deferred,* tenBroek and Matson describe why early educators of blind people saw the need to separate schools from workshops. Sheltered workshops for blind people continue to be a major source of contention between blind workers and their leaders and the agencies sponsoring them. For the worker, it was a dead end and meant permanent dependency. "The Volunteers of America, an offshoot of the Salvation Army, currently sponsors at least 70 such workshops; while perhaps the most successful of all the mission or church-sponsored workshop chains is that of the Goodwill Industries, founded by a Methodist minister in 1905, which by 1957 controlled 120 shops throughout the country" (Matson, 1990, p. 753). Early hospitals, also under religious auspices, took care of paupers, the disabled and the insane. The workhouse, or almshouse, evolved from the Poor Laws of Elizabethan England and required labor for welfare assistance. "The workhouse provided an institutionalized form of poor relief; and in keeping with Elizabethan assumptions of the characterological causes of poverty, it was made as disagreeable as possible and its wages held to a bare minimum above starvation so that not many would willingly seek admission or contentedly remain" (p. 754). Finally, the sheltered workshops in the United States were also associated with the early efforts in the 19th century to establish schools for the blind. As previously noted, early educators of the blind believed that education and employment needed to be separated. In 1962, Professor Jacobus tenBroek, a nationally recognized expert on welfare policy, commented on the debate concerning the proper function of sheltered workshops.

> The institution of the sheltered workshop, for over a century an inconspicuous feature of the American welfare scene, has recently emerged from its obscurity to become the storm-center of one of the liveliest controversies in the entire field of social work and public welfare. At the heart of the controversy is a fundamental disagreement over the proper function and future role of the sheltered shop. One viewpoint holds that a proper role of the shops is that of providing work evaluation, determination of abilities, and the development of work tolerance on the part of disabled persons—along with vocational training itself—as part of the process of vocational rehabilitation. More recently, doctors and health officials have begun to campaign for the use of the workshop as a medical facility for restorative, adjustive and pre-vocational services centering around the principle of work therapy. Finally, the oldest and perhaps still the most widely held viewpoint is that which regards the workshop as a place of remunerative employment for disabled individuals.
>
> Two of these approaches to the sheltered workshop find support for their arguments in federal law and administrative rulings. The proponents of the vocational adjustment and training function point out that, since the passage of the Vocational Rehabilitaiton Act in 1954, sheltered workshops have been recognized as a legitimate training adjunct of the federal-state vocational rehabilitation program; and in addition they may cite the majority ruling of the National Labor Relations Board, handed down in March of this year, (1960), that rehabilitation is *the* essential function of the workshop.
>
> The defenders of the employment status of the workshop may demonstrate that, even with the Vocational Rehabilitation Act, "sheltered workshop" is defined as primarily a place which provides remunerative employment, and

that in fact rehabilitation administrators frequently regard the placement of their clients in such shops as sufficient to meet the remunerative placement of their clients' requirements which are the ultimate objective of vocational rehabilitation programs. Moreover, the employment argument finds further support in the fact that the very exemption of sheltered workshops from the minimum wage provisions of the Fair Labor Standards Act was granted on the premise that they are places of employment.

To some extent the issues raised by these differences of viewpoint are theoretical in nature, involving such questions as: What are the proper goals of workshops? What is their greatest usefulness as instruments of welfare? (tenBroek, 1962, p. 19–20)

Gradually the treatment of blind workers in sheltered workshops became a major concern of the organized blind movement. Workers themselves, as well as many other blind people, either experienced directly or saw the contradictions embodied in employment in sheltered workshops. By 1950, they saw such employment as being neither ennobling nor leading toward competitive employment. The National Federation of the Blind sought at least the minimum wage for workshop employees, and raised questions about upward mobility for blind workers and under-representation of blind workers at any level above the bottom. It sought the right of blind workers to organize themselves in labor movements and to bargain collectively with management. The struggle has continued for more than four decades, one workshop at a time. Some workshops have voluntarily responded to some concerns, such as the minimum wage, but in most cases, picketing, litigation, and governmental intervention were necessary before improvements occurred.

James Gashel reviewed several criticisms of sheltered workshops in his March 26, 1986, testimony before the Committee on Small Business of the United States Senate. In addition to arguing for collective bargaining for blind employees, he presented evidence of economic exploitation and a lack of mobility opportunity.

A description of a typical sheltered workshop might help to set a framework for the recommended changes we intend to offer for S. 2147. Our specimen workshop is the Industries Program for the Blind and Handicapped operated by the State of Connecticut, Board of Education and Services for the Blind. The workshop has plant locations in Newington and Wethersfield. Both will soon merge into a single facility located in West Hartford. The figures I will cite concerning employment and pay come from 1983 and represent the pattern of this program's operation in the years before and since.

If you include all positions from direct labor to top management in the Connecticut workshop, there is a total workforce of 116 individuals. Eighty-five perform direct labor jobs, and 31 hold positions classified as management, supervision, and indirect labor. Of the 85 direct labor workers, only 6 are sighted with no reported handicaps. Eight sighted workers have handicaps, and the remaining 71 direct labor employees are blind, some with other handicaps. As for the 31 employees classified as management, supervision, or indirect labor, 20 of them are sighted without reported handicaps. Six more are sighted with handicaps, and 5 are blind—3 with other handicaps and 2 without.

Ninety-three percent of the employees in direct labor positions are individuals reported to be blind or handicapped. But in the management, supervision, and indirect labor category, blind and handicapped people represent only 35% of the work force. These, of course, are the better paying jobs. The figures bear that out. Total direct labor pay amounts to $151,424, divided up among 85 employees (93% of whom are blind or handicapped). By contrast, pay to managers, supervisors, and indirect labor workers amounts to $293,597, divided up among 31 employees (only 35% of whom are blind or handicapped).

As for hourly pay averages, all blind and handicapped direct labor workers combined earn an average of $2.04 per hour, whereas all sighted handicapped or nonhandicapped direct labor workers earn an average of $4.09 per hour. Sighted workers without handicaps earn $4.20 per hour. As for managers and supervisors, sighted people without handicaps (who are in the majority in this category, holding 20 out of 31 positions) earn an average of $8.25 per hour, in comparison to their blind and handicapped co-workers, who earn an average of $5.54 per hour.

Now for the bottom line: total pay to all 116 employees at the Connecticut workshop is $445,021. There are 26 sighted employees who do not have handicaps, representing 22.41% of the work force. Yet these 26 individuals were paid $283,911, or 63.79% of the total pay for the Connecticut workshop. That leaves $161,110 to be paid to blind or handicapped workers, or a little over 36% of the total pay. But the blind and handicapped (who according to these figures received a little over 36% of the pay) represented almost 78% of the work force. Pay levels in the Connecticut workshop seem to depend strictly upon the extent of a person's handicap or blindness. The best jobs and the best pay go to sighted individuals who do not have handicaps. (pp. 256–257)

Blind employees have used strikes and otherwise confronted management in several workshops in Tennessee, Ohio, Illinois, Texas, Arkansas, and other states (Hodge, 1989). While blind employees have asked for minimum wage, competitive employment opportunities, union representation, and management opportunities, workshop managers usually have argued economic necessity or justified low wages in terms of the special problems of blind workers. Charles Brown described similar conditions in the Virginia Industries for the Blind which were typified in a recent nationally publicized strike at a sheltered workshop in Lubbock, Texas.

LUBBOCK, Texas (AP)—Blind employees at a workshop established to rehabilitate them say they're being exploited and are demanding the same wages their sighted counterparts get for comparable work.

But the founder of the Southwest Lighthouse for the Blind says the workshop trains blind people for work in the private sector and is not required to pay the minimum wage.

The U.S. Department of Labor is investigating the workshop's wages, and Lighthouse officials are to appear next month before an administrative law judge to defend the separate wage scales for blind and sighted employees.

"I think they're trying to have more of a factory out there than to do something for the blind," said David Rocco, a former Lighthouse employee who led a workers' strike in August and was laid off in January.

The dispute comes at a time when the blind are increasingly questioning their treatment at such organizations. About 100 similar workshops employ 6,000 visually impaired people nation wide. Employees at workshops in Houston and Cincinnati have formed unions in the wake of wage and labor disputes. Unionization efforts by workers in Little Rock, Arkansas, were denied by an appeals court.

"Blind people have been exploited in workshops since workshops came into being," said James Gashel, Director of Governmental Affairs for the National Federation of the Blind in Baltimore.

"When you're paying $2.10 an hour, you're going to have a lot of wage disputes," added the Federation's President, Marc Maurer. "It's not enough to live on."

In Lubbock fourteen blind workers, carrying canes and wearing signs reading "Lighthouse wages are from the Dark Ages," walked off their jobs in August to protest the $2.05 hourly wage and their $65-a-month health insurance fee.

They want the Lighthouse to pay them the same $3.35 minimum wage other employees receive. (*Columbia Daily Tribune*, March 6, 1989)

More than forty articles have appeared in the *Braille Monitor* since 1970 describing discrimination, exploitation, or alleged intimidation. The intensity of the conflict is perhaps reflected in the following statement of the journal's editor: "It is no exaggeration to say that the term 'professional,' which should be positive and complimentary when applied to employees of programs that are designed to give service to people, has become to the blind of this country a virtual swear word—a bitter term of mockery and disillusionment" (Jernigan, 1988a, p. 228).

Workshops have grown in both size and numbers. They have large budgets, represent large community resources, and provide relatively desirable incomes for management. Workshops have a national organization to lobby for their interests and receive preferred treatment from governmental agencies. They offer for their managers, status, middle-class employment, and long term employment prospects. Hence, workshops represent a resource, control of which is carefully guarded by management.

Goal Displacement

Scott (1967) studied changes that occurred in the management of sheltered workshops and illustrated how organizational interests created conditions frequently seen as contrary to the interest of blind workers. In the early decades of this century, workers for the blind consistently argued that work was ennobling and that blind people should be integrated into the community through work relationships. However, as sheltered workshops became larger, marketing and management skills, exceeding those routinely available, were required. Engineering, safety, and concerns about economic viability led to managers who were guided by commercial, rather than social service standards.

Scott used the concept of "goal displacement" to describe the tendency of the "day-to-day policy decisions of an organization to modify, transform, and occasionally even to subvert the objectives for which the organization was established." He presented as evidence several statements from annual meetings of the American Association of Workers for the Blind. A survey of twenty-five workshop managers in 1935 concluded that it was undesirable to employ new blind workers above age forty-five. "When we take into consideration the months and even years that it takes to train a blind person to be a top notch producer, we realize that any higher age limit would tend to reduce the years of usefulness to such an extent that it might well be a losing proposition" (AAWB Proceedings, 1935, p. 83).

Organizational maintenance and budgetary concerns cannot explain the intensity of the resistance of many workshop managers to worker's concerns. There are now too many economically viable workshops which pay more than the minimum wage and which bargain with the workers for this to be a valid explanation. Some managers and their boards of directors are simply unwilling to concede any power or economic improvement to blind workers. "Regardless of institutional affiliation, the director of a rehabilitation program is accountable to multiple public, private and corporate constituencies as never before" (Albrecht, 1992, p. 189).

Developing a New Profession

Workers for the blind have openly attempted to professionalize themselves for the last fifty years. As I have indicated in Chapter 2, this process is best understood in terms of the economic privilege and power which have resulted for those occupational groups to whom the wider society accords professional recognition. "As professionalizing occupations move to create and affirm collective worth, one of the incentives for participation, as well as one of the major goals of the movement, is to secure the supports for individual dignity and individual careers" (Larson, 1977, p. 157). In this section I will review the growth of occupational organizations which merged into the groups that currently claim professional status and examine some of the conflicts which have resulted from several aspects of this professionalizing process.

By 1910, employment in the field of working with blind people was dominated by two organizations—the American Association of Workers for the Blind (AAWB) and the American Association of Instructors of the Blind (AAIB). The AAIB, founded in 1871, was primarily comprised of educators of the blind. The American Association of Workers for the Blind, founded in 1905, was a more broadly based organization. Agenda items at the 1905 meeting included industrial education, employment, standardization of a tactual reading system, the welfare of elderly blind persons, boarding homes and other housing arrangements for blind adults, nurseries for blind babies, and home teaching services for adults. Frequently, members of the more prestigious AAIB also belonged to the AAWB (Koestler, 1976).

Additional impetus for this new employment arena came in 1920 when President Wilson signed the Smith-Fess Act, which led to a $750,000 appropriation in 1921 for a joint federal-state program of vocational rehabilitation for the physically handicapped. Thus began the flow of federal money which has become a major economic resource for the blindness rehabilitation industry. In part, this legislation reflected a broad base of concern for blinded World War I veterans, and the establishment of the Federal Board of Vocational Education has gradually led to the jointly funded federal-state rehabilitation program of today. This program, currently supported by 80 percent federal and 20 percent matching state funds, has operated since 1921 without ever being subject to significant legislative opposition.

The AAIB and AAWB conducted separate biennial conventions in alternate years. In 1921 the AAWB considered an item which had been discussed in 1920 at the AAIB convention concerning the need for a national foundation to provide leadership in work with or for blind people. The conferees, representing all major employee groups, unanimously approved by-laws establishing the American Foundation for the Blind. This new organization was to fulfill the convention hope "that there should be in work for the blind some sort of General Foundation representative of and responsive to every important phase or branch of the profession." (Koestler, 1976, p. 19) The future American Foundation for the Blind would have three main bureaus: the Bureau of Information and Publicity, to collect and disseminate information about blindness; the Bureau of Research, to fund and conduct research about blindness; and the Bureau of Education, to promote all aspects regarding the education of blind people. The AFB, through successful fund-raising efforts, including the involvement of Helen Keller, became a significant resource for the developing professions in work with the blind.

> In 1920, in arguing for the need for a national agency or foundation, one prominent leader, L. W. Wallace, director of the Red Cross Institute for the Blind, commented, the possibilities of vocational activity for the blind will never be realized until there is a change of attitude on the part of many of the blind themselves. . . . The attitude that many of the blind assume or acquire, or it may be a part of their natural psychology, is one of the greatest drawbacks to their development and opportunity. What do I mean? It is this, they are supersensitive, critical, and unappreciative (as reported by Koestler, 1976, p. 21).

It would not be many years until a national organization of blind people would develop a philosophy about blindness which frequently conflicted with the claims about blindness made by many professionals.

Public and private support for rehabilitation programs for blind people continued to grow in the 1930s. Public appropriations grew even faster after World War II, when more than sixteen thousand newly blinded veterans returned home. Robert Irwin, nationally prominent as head of the American Foundation for the Blind, focused attention on the specialized nature of work for the blind in "Why Rehabilitation of the Blind is the Function of a Special Agency for the Blind" (1943). Because of the severity of the handicaps of blind people, their rehabilitation was more difficult and called for agencies specializing in services to the blind.

> Because blindness affects all phases of an individual's life—even such simple matters as eating, dressing, reading one's personal mail, walking down the

street alone—and also because the psychological effects of blindness are probably more severe than for any other type of physical handicap, vocational rehabilitation of the blind is as much a matter of social case work as it is of vocational training and placement. Therefore the rehabilitation of the blind is more appropriately a function of a social agency, such as the commission for the blind or the department of welfare, than of a department of education. (Irwin, 1943)

Koestler, (1976) wrote that the decade of the 1950's was one of expanding opportunities for blind people. However, to access these opportunities, the blind had to travel farther from home and to do so independently. During this decade, many workers for the blind concluded that a new specialty was needed. Older generation mobility instructors, who had frequently been blind themselves, were not judged adequate for the current travel demands.

A New Specialization

In 1953 Father Thomas J. Carroll called a meeting of experts at his agency in Massachusetts to discuss the need for a new occupational specialization. "The occasion for the conference, the invitees were informed, was 'the increasing recognition of the danger involved in allowing untrained persons to set themselves up as [mobility] experts'" (Koestler, 1976, p. 317).

In 1958 the Federal Office of Rehabilitation, directed by Mr. Louis Rives, adopted as a program priority the training of mobility instructors. The American Foundation for the Blind was given a grant to convene a national conference of experts to define this new specialization. The first step toward the professionalization of this area was taken, according to Koestler, with the recommendation that one year of specialized graduate education be required for mobility instructors.

> The conferees also came out firmly, although not unanimously, with what they knew would be an inflammatory stand: that "the teaching of mobility was a task of a sighted, rather than a blind, individual." The concept of the blind mobility instructor was "bankrupt," the majority insisted, if only because that instructor was just as incapable of seeing danger as his trainee, and was therefore unable to protect the latter in a hazardous situation (pp. 317–318).

By now blindness rehabilitation had attracted federal funding and had appeared on several university campuses. For reasons I have not been able to document, masters degrees in blindness rehabilitation were generally not available at universities of major academic stature. However, work for the blind had found an additional institutional base to legitimate itself. It could now produce research and further buttress claims of expertise. "The professionals acquired not only an institutional basis on which to develop and standardize knowledge and technologies; they also received, in university training, a most powerful legitimation for their claims to cognitive and technical superiority and to social and economic benefits" (Larson, 1977, p. 136). This approach was challenged by blind consumers, as well as by blind and sighted agency personnel. Opponents cited discrimination and ignorance about the capabilities of blind travelers. To many, this issue symbolized "featherbedding" and professional behavior contrary to goals and philosophies of rehabilitation. The debate is reflected, for example, in articles or responses by Carl Olson (1981) and others.

Olson, at that time a staff member of Nebraska Services for the Visually Impaired, focused on the self-interest of this new professional subgroup as the major source of the certification of orientation and mobility specialists. He noted that this new certification would enhance employment opportunities for university-based professionals: "The claim that the teaching of this fundamental skill is an art and that training at the graduate level is required in order to practice the art, we regard as nothing more than self-serving rhetoric on the part of the O & M establishment, aimed at enhancing the professional status of O & M practitioners" (p. 338).

Despite the intensity of the opposition, blind people were removed from this area of professionally licensed competitive employment. The AAWB and its successor organization, the Association for the Education and Rehabilitation of the Blind and Visually Impaired (AER), formalized the certification of mobility instructors. Only sighted persons with one year of specialized graduate instruction were to be certified, and such requirements were accepted by many private agencies. However, certification requirements have not been imposed by most state-funded agencies. People with such credentials are either unavailable or judged to be no more competent than non-licensed individuals. Sometimes the requirement is rejected because it is considered to be discriminatory.

This issue illustrates one source of conflict within the occupational group itself. The licensing and accreditation requirements are most frequently utilized in smaller and privately funded agencies. Consumers have less leverage in these agencies partly because the boards of directors are comprised of wealthy or prominent citizens who usually know little about the issues involved. On the other hand, those who work in the larger state-funded rehabilitation programs illustrate the influence of the publicly funded and bureaucratically organized work setting. Consumer groups can directly lobby state and federal politicians. Funding can be threatened and laws against discrimination can be invoked. In this context, the requirement that mobility instructors have a master's degree is not worth fighting about for the administrators involved. For example, the director of the Missouri Rehabilitation Services for the Blind does not consider the AER license requirements necessary for the employment of mobility instructors. "We consider applicants for positions on the basis of ability, training and education—not on their visual acuity" (Vogel, 1992).

If a blind person can travel independently with a long white cane or guide dog, a properly trained blind or partially sighted man or woman can surely teach another. If a particularly dangerous situation is involved, alternative sources of visual information can be used when judged necessary by the instructor. To say that no blind individual, regardless of competence and level of education, can ever be certified as an orientation and mobility instructor, in my opinion, is discrimination, plain and simple. In addition, publicly mandated and funded service programs are in a most awkward position if, for example, they cannot offer mobility instruction to clients because there is a shortage of certified, sighted mobility instructors with master's degrees (Vogel 1992).

Fewer than ten of the fifty state agencies even bother to participate in the accreditation process of the National Accreditation Council of Agencies Serving the Blind and Visually Handicapped. However, the certification requirement and accreditation process are strongly supported by the leadership of the largest organization of workers for the blind—the Association for the Education and Rehabilitation of the Blind and Visually Impaired.

Support from the federal government was given to the American Foundation for the Blind with the intention of promoting the agenda of interested personnel. Such conferences then legitimated demands for graduate educational centers to train these new specialists. The new educational centers then obtained federal funding to help deal with this newly discovered manpower need. Subsequently, the endowment of the AFB was becoming large enough, and its fund-raising successful enough, that it did not always require government or other foundation funding for agenda-setting conferences it sponsored.

Societies institutionalize expertise through occupational groups recognized as professions, and then specialized esoteric knowledge is applied to individual cases. "Experts were organized in collegial groups which included mutual respect for claims of occupational expertise. Specialized training schools, licensure and codes of ethics were thought to bring benefits to both the professional and the client" (Abbott, 1988, p. 5). As I indicated in Chapter 5, scientific discourse created images about blindness that identified blind people as significantly different from the sighted. In addition, the medical model of deviance was almost always referred to when discussing the blind person. Something was wrong that could be fixed if the blind person accepted his/her condition and the help of experts. The condition could not be removed, but under the proper instruction of experts, individuals could become better adjusted to their blindness. The definitions of blindness were almost always catastrophic. Conflict became intense when many blind people sought a new definition of blindness to replace the harmful one being created by some agencies and many of their professional workers and researchers. As Friedson (1970) observed, "A profession is distinct from other occupations in that it has been given the right to control its own work" (pp. 71–72). Evaluation by others outside the profession is seen as intolerable and illegitimate.

Meanwhile, consumers argued that the interpretations of blindness were not the sole domain of specialists or professionals. Blind people were as ordinary and varied as other members of the general population. Blindness was not a mysterious or profoundly complex situation. One of the first "professional" responses rejecting this consumer point of view was an article, "Who Says Blindness is Just an Inconvenience?" by Paul Schulz (1977). Schulz argued that equating blindness with inconvenience was wrong, and that to do so was a defense mechanism of denial. Individuals who denied the severity of blindness had not fully matured. "For some persons, however, it is a mechanism they retain for a lifetime because they have never developed a more mature way of coping with a harsh reality or with their perception of such reality. If an experience is too difficult to handle or too painful to accept, they deny the reality of either the physical or the emotional fact" (p. 230). For Schulz, sight is the best sense receptor and most effective means of gaining information about the environment. Its absence is much more than an inconvenience. The loss is serious; sight has no equivalent. "If an individual loses an arm, a leg, or through paralysis the function of any part of the body, the loss is serious, and adaptation to life without it is nearly always difficult and emotionally painful" (p. 230).

Other professionals continued this argument, focusing on the importance of professional services. Mentioned above as instrumental in the movement toward certification of mobility instructors, Louis Rives, president of the National Accreditation Council of Agencies Serving the Blind and Visually Handicapped, proclaimed at the 1977 annual meeting of NAC "that any thinking blind person who considers the matter objectively and reasonably knows that blindness is a severe disability because the whole world is predicated on seeing things" (p. 9). Most blind people need all the professional skills that can be brought to bear. "There are only two ways in which you can make blind people and sighted people absolutely equal. One of them is to restore the sight of all the blind people. And the other one is to pluck the eyes out of all the rest of the world. And neither one of these things is going to happen in our time" (p. 9).

Similar statements evoked many rebuttals, including several published in the *Journal of Visual Impairment and Blindness*. Anthony Cobb (1977) argued that Schulz misrepresented and oversimplified the consumer arguments.

> To say that blindness is always just an inconvenience to every blind person would be as much nonsense as is the notion that it is inevitably tragic. What Jernigan has repeatedly voiced is that with training and opportunity blindness can be reduced to the level of a physical inconvenience much as can excessive height or weight, awkwardness, lefthandedness, or other physical characteristics which deviate to some degree from the norm (pp. 406–407).

As opposed to the "blindness establishment," Cobb linked his defense of consumerism with "progressive agencies."

Carl Olson (1977) observed that Schulz had discussed blindness strictly in terms of psychological categories.

> Perhaps even Schulz would agree that many people who claim that their blindness has been reduced to an inconvenience are successful and competent individuals. I know many such individuals, and I find in them no evidence of maladjustment. If Schulz chooses to characterize the attitude which these competent and well-adjusted people have toward blindness as an immature and inappropriate response to a harsh reality, I would say that his position is grounded in something other than sound reasoning and scientific observation (p. 406).

For Olson, blindness is not a tragedy because art masterpieces cannot be observed in detail. Most people never see them, much less in their detail.

Schulz had observed that it was more than an irritation when a blind pedestrian was struck by an automobile. Olson responded that properly trained blind people are being hit by automobiles at no greater rate than anyone else.

> In speaking of the disadvantages of blindness the important thing to emphasize is that blindness does not entail the loss of any value which is essential to human happiness and fulfillment. If it did, then that would be tragic. But when one compares the sort of "deprivations" which Schulz mentions (art masterpieces and delicate facial features) with such human values as independence, self-esteem, the love and respect of one's fellows, etc., they are surely more on the order of annoyances and inconveniences than tragedies and calamities. (p. 407)

Several articles appeared in the *Braille Monitor* in the decades of the 1960s and 70s arguing for a reinterpretation of the meaning and significance of blindness. Writers maintained that blind people are little different from others—except with regards to sight. Alternative sensory information is always available, and experience, appropriate education, and opportunity bring more and more of it. Blindness need not be traumatic. Unfortunately, people learn to accept definitions of blindness which, when internalized, become quite limiting. However, with a proper outlook and the right education and opportunity, one could reduce his or her blindness to a nuisance or inconvenience. Such arguments are typified in Jernigan's 1982 article entitled "Blindness—Handicap or Characteristic," in which he comments on "catastrophic" definitions of blindness.

> According to this view what the blind person needs most is not travel training but therapy. He will be taught to accept his limitations as insurmountable and his difference from others as unbridgeable. He will be encouraged to adjust to his painful station as a second-class citizen and discouraged from any thought of breaking and entering the first-class compartment. Moreover, all of this will be done in the name of teaching him "independence" and a "realistic" approach to his blindness. (1982a, p. 496)

Professional Interests Versus Consumer Interests

Independence, self-reliance, and competitive employment are among the goals of major consumer organizations of handicapped people. The goals of the organized blind in terms of legislative efforts, self-help, education of the public, and programs to engender self-efficacy are congruent with rehabilitation goals. Yet, as this chapter has shown, a deep and growing conflict absorbs much human energy and organizational resources. In addition to picketing, lobbying, initiating lawsuits and other forms of confrontation, consumers are questioning the very assumptions about blindness held by those who provide services.

Regrettably and predictably, the leadership of many agencies and professional organizations resist consumer participation. In *Professions and Power,* Johnson (1967) noted that the political dimensions of professions do not always reflect disembodied societal needs. Instead, they sometimes impose services and definitions of problems on individual clients. In complex societies, blind and other handicapped people are labeled as deviants and special organizations and professions develop to handle the newly defined social problem (Freidson, 1965; Gubrium, 1986; Gusfield, 1984). Such programs are organized bureaucratically. Social welfare and educational activities alike embody differential power in relationships between the participants. As representatives of the organized structure of power, social service personnel are employees dependent upon the on-going processes of the organization for their livelihood. There are few employment alternatives except at similar highly specialized bureaucratic agencies. Consequently, there is a powerful force, as Weber noted, for agency personnel to become extensions of the inherent power arrangements.

The social implications of the bureaucratic process include the defense of vested interests by those having greater power, the social control and domination of subordinates by superordinates, the specialization of work and related claims of expertise, and a refined and developed rhetoric justifying the entire process. The defense of vested interests and the control of subordinates is well illustrated in the thorough study of the conditions in a New York hospital for retarded children by Rothman and Rothman (1984).

In the social constructionist tradition of research on deviance, Joseph Gusfield (1984) describes the social process by which professionals lay claim to and seek public support for their work.

> The sense of mission about the solution to exigent problems has been a significant ingredient in the actions of practitioners and partisans. It has been built on a belief in the certainty that the problem actually exists, that it is of major proportions, and that the work of the program or the movement can help in resolving it. It involves a theory and a body of presumed fact, both of which are assured. Such theories and facts are not neutral matters, a point of view held in an academic seminar. They constitute vital sources for a sense of professional esteem, client respect, and

the ability to maintain legitimate occupational place. They constitute the source of belief that a knowledge base has been buttressed by the methods and expertise of scientific and technical professionals (p. 44).

In "work for the blind," many professional organizations, most large private agencies, many schools for the blind, the few university training centers, and the American Foundation for the Blind frequently demonstrate similar and often coordinated responses to consumer criticisms. Their representatives are involved in developing agendas for national conferences and promote the professional interests of their field. As this chapter has documented, funding moves from public resources to private agencies which then legitimate demands for additional funding for yet more educational and research efforts.

Many blind people, particularly those in accord with the philosophy and programs of the National Federation of the Blind, now reject programs they judge to be paternalistic, demeaning, dependency creating, and otherwise harmful. They reject token participation of consumers in programs or agencies that provide services. As consumer political effectiveness continues to grow, the threat to the funding and public legitimacy of existing programs may result in a change in attitudes toward consumer participation and definitions of blindness.

In the following speech, Kenneth Jernigan, then President of the National Federation of the Blind, focused on problems in the blindness system. He analyzes conflicts between agencies and professionals and the consumer movement. He argues that the support of blind people, through their democratically elected organizations, is crucial for both improving and preserving the "blindness system."

CONSUMERISM:
IMPROVING THE SERVICE DELIVERY SYSTEM

Today we are talking about consumerism. The fact that we are, along with the popularity and recurrence of the theme, means that there is a felt need and that there are problems. In the summer of 1988 I participated in a panel discussion on this topic at the AER convention in Montreal. Some of the things which I said at the time bear repeating, for they deal with basic questions—matters concerning relationships and performance in our field.

At the National Federation of the Blind convention in Chicago in

1988, 2,443 people registered as attendees. No other group has that kind of attendance. You know it, and I know it. In October of 1989 the National Federation of the Blind distributed (on cassette, on flexible disc, in Braille, and in print) over 29,000 copies of its magazine the *Braille Monitor*. Again, no other publication in our field has that kind of circulation, or anything even approaching it.

At my first NFB convention in 1952 barely 150 people were present, and we had no monthly publication. At that 1952 convention we spent more than fifty percent of our time talking about the rehabilitation system—what it was doing, how to improve it, and what we wanted from it. At our 1988 convention we had twenty-five hours of program content, and we spent a total of forty-five minutes (or three percent of the time) dealing with the rehabilitation system of the United States. Of that forty-five minutes, fifteen minutes was spent hearing from the federal Rehabilitation Commissioner; fifteen minutes was spent hearing from our Director of Governmental Affairs, who talked about problems blind people were having with the system; and the final fifteen minutes was spent with questions and comments from the audience, indicating their concern with the failure of the system to deliver. In short, only one percent of the program time was used to hear from the rehabilitation system, and none of the time was spent talking about threats to the system or how to save it. Why?

Is it simply, as some have charged, that the members of the Federation (all of the thousands and tens of thousands of them—or, at least, their leaders) are negative and destructive—irresponsible radicals and agency haters? No. Such a thesis cannot be sustained. The facts do not support it. Let us turn again to the statistics of the 1988 NFB convention.

Kurt Cylke, head of the National Library Service for the Blind and Physically Handicapped, was with us for the entire week, and so were several of his staff. Day after day they answered questions, talked with our members, and planned with us for the future. There was an atmosphere of partnership and mutual trust.

Likewise, top officials of the Social Security Administration were present to speak and participate. The Deputy Commissioner for Policy and External Affairs had a forty-minute segment on the program, and other Social Security personnel conducted a seminar and answered questions for most of an afternoon. As with the Library, there was no tension or confrontation—only partnership and a feeling of shared interest and mutual concern. Moreover, with Social Security it must be remembered that many blind people throughout the country experience problems with underpayments, demands for return of overpayments, denial of applications, and similar difficulties; and more often than not, the National Federation of the Blind represents those blind persons in hearings to reverse Social Security's actions. Millions of dollars and numerous professional judgments are repeatedly called into question. Yet, there is no hostility—only friendliness and joint effort. On a continuing basis the National Federation of the Blind and the Social Security Administration share information, exchange ideas, and work together in a spirit of cooperative harmony.

In short, our problems come only with the rehabilitation system, with some of the private agencies which function as part of that system, and with a group of educators. And even here there must be a further narrowing and focusing, for the problem is with the system itself and some of its more vocal spokespersons, not with all of its component parts or personnel. An increasing number of those in the system are beginning to take a new look and work with us. The very fact of our discussion here this morning is an evidence of that trend and the shift in thinking.

This brings me to our topic, "Consumerism," I think blind people must have not an exclusive but a major role in shaping the blindness system. Otherwise, the system will die. Moreover, when I say "blind people," I do not mean just blind individuals. I mean democratic membership organizations *of* the blind. I mean effective participation by the blind, and the only way that can be achieved is through organizations of the blind. In a sense, of course, blind people have always shaped the system, as indeed they do today. In most cases blind persons started (or played a major part in starting) the agencies. There have always been blind agency directors, and individual blind persons prominent in the community have from the beginning served on advisory and policy boards and lent their names and prestige to funding and public support.

Even so, the system has traditionally been custodial in nature and highhanded in dealing with meaningful input from the blind. This is why the system is in trouble. It is in danger of being absorbed into generic programs for the disabled, starving for lack of funds, and losing its position of centrality and perceived importance in the lives of the blind. This would not be the case if the average, thinking, responsible blind adult in this country felt that the system really mattered—excluding, of course, the blind people who work in the system.

Let me be clearly understood. I am not saying that rehabilitation, training in mobility, assistance for the newly blind, or education are not important—urgently important; for they are. Rather, I am saying that year by year more and more blind persons have come to feel that the system is not effectively providing those things and that it is both unresponsive and irrelevant. Remember that I am talking about the system as a whole, not individual agencies or particular people working in those agencies.

It is not, as a few have claimed, that the organized blind wish to take control of the agencies. It is, from the point of view of the system, far worse than that. It is that more and more blind people are coming to feel that, in the things that count in their daily lives, what the agencies have to offer won't help and doesn't matter.

If I felt that the system was hopeless and that nothing could or should be done to improve it, I would not be here today talking with you. It is late, but if honest evaluation and forthright action occur, I think the system can be saved—and that it is worth saving.

However, certain things must be said without equivocation. As a beginning, the agencies must change their attitudes about criticism and about the role of the organized blind in decision making. The matter of Fred Schroeder is a case in point. As most members of this organization know, Mr. Schroeder is blind. He is currently Director of the New Mexico Commission for the Blind. Before taking that job, he taught mobility professionally, received all of the academic credentials for doing so, and then was denied certification by this organization (the Association for Education and Rehabilitation of the Blind and Visually Impaired). The denial was based on the belief that a blind person cannot safely and competently teach another blind person how to travel—or, if you like, teach another blind person mobility. The National Federation of the Blind as an organization and I as an individual thought you were wrong in that decision, and we were entitled to that opinion. On the other hand, it was perfectly proper for your organization to believe that you were right to attack our position, but it was not proper for the members of your organization to attack us (as some of you did) on irrelevant grounds—denigrating our character and morals because of our beliefs. Of course, the same would pertain for our treatment of you.

Moreover, workers in the blindness system must resist the growing tendency to hide behind the term "professionalism" and must stop treating "professionalism" as if it were a sacred mystery. There is a teachable body of knowledge which can be learned about giving service to the blind; but much of that knowledge is a matter of common sense, good judgment, and experience. Most thinking blind persons (certainly those who have been blind for any length of time and have had any degree of success) know at least as much about what they and other blind people want and need from the system as the professionals do, and it must also be kept in mind that not every act of a "professional" is necessarily a "professional" act or based on "professionalism." Just as in other fields in America today, the professionals in the blindness system must be judged on their behavior and not merely their credentials.

Consider, for instance, the question of whether children with residual vision should be taught Braille. After careful consideration the members of the National Federation of the Blind believe that every such child should at least have the option of being taught Braille. Some of the educators (especially those who cannot fluently read and write Braille) resist this view. Is their opinion a "professional" judgement, or is it a decision based on vested interest? Whichever it is, the views of the organized blind are entitled to serious consideration and not simply a brush-off, with the statement that the blind don't know what they are talking about and that they probably have bad motives and morals into the bargain.

This brings me back to what I said about Kurt Cylke and the National Library Service for the Blind and Physically Handicapped. The libraries are not in trouble, and (regardless of economic conditions or changing theories) the libraries won't be in trouble. They won't because the blind of this country won't let it happen. And, yes, we have the power to give substance to our feeling. We don't control Kurt Cylke or the libraries. We don't want to—and besides, he wouldn't permit it. Neither does he control us—and for the same reasons. We support the National Library Service for the Blind and Physically Handicapped because we need it, because it gives useful and good service, and because its leaders understand that they *exist* to give us service, and that they have accountability to us. What I have said about the Library is also true of the Social Security Administration and an increasing number of agencies and individuals in the fields of rehabilitation and education.

But the hard core of the blindness system still resists, to its detriment and ours. It tries to say that it speaks for the blind because the head of an agency is blind or because blind people serve on a staff or board. No great intellect is required to understand that in a representative democracy only those elected *by* a group can speak *for* that group; that the heads of agencies can have vested interests which transcend their blindness; and that when an agency can pick and choose individual blind spokespersons from the community, it can get people who will say whatever it wants them to say.

Unless things change, I believe the central core of the blindness system will sink into obscurity and wither away, but I believe this need not happen and should not happen. Blind people (and that means the organized blind) must have a major voice in shaping the blindness system and programs which operate within it—whether those programs be sheltered shops, residential schools, state agencies, or private nonprofit organizations. It must be a partnership—and not a partnership of dominance and subservience but of consenting equals—a partnership based on trust, respect, and mutuality. Let these things happen, and all else will follow. Let these things happen, and the system will thrive.

If those who work in the public and private agencies want broad support from the blind community, they must be responsive to the concerns which the blind perceive as important. Today there are relatively few major issues which divide the organized blind and the agencies. Twenty years ago it appeared (at least, on the surface) that there was at least one such issue—the National Accreditation Council for Agencies Serving the Blind and Visually Handicapped (NAC). But the problem was more apparent than real. NAC (despite its few remaining vocal supporters) has never been a significant factor in the lives of the nation's blind and is now rapidly becoming a dead letter and a subject only for the historians. It has never been able to get more than twenty or twenty-five percent of the nation's eligible agencies to accept its accreditation, and increasingly as the larger and more prominent agencies have pulled away from it, it has been forced to try to keep its numbers up by accrediting smaller and less well known organizations. Let the dead be dead, and let the rest of us move on to better things.

The real question we face is not how to resolve controversies between consumers and the agencies but whether consumers can continue to feel that the agencies on balance are relevant enough and important enough for the consumers to nurture and save them—in short, whether there can be common cause, shared purpose, mutual respect, and true partnership. Certainly the problems which face us are formidable and challenging. We still have a long way to go in improving the climate of public opinions so that the blind can have opportunity and full access to the main channels of everyday life. We have made tremendous progress in this area, but much yet remains to be done. All other things being equal, the job can best be handled through joint effort by the blind and the agencies, but handled it must be whether the agencies participate or not.

Likewise, there is a broad spectrum of specific programs and activities, ranging from technology to education to employment, which need urgent and sustained attention—and again (all other things being equal) the job can best be handled by joint effort on the part of the blind community and the agencies. But one way or another, the blind intend to achieve full equality and first class status in society. The question is what part the agencies will play and what relationship they will have with the increasingly powerful consumer movement.

The story is told that one evening a nightclub patron approached the bandstand and said to the drummer, "Does your dog bite?"

"No," the drummer said, "he doesn't."

The man reached down to pet the dog, and it almost bit his arm off. He leaped back in a fury and said to the drummer, "I thought you said your dog didn't bite."

"He doesn't," the drummer said, "but that isn't my dog."

You see, the man asked the wrong question, so he got an unsatisfactory answer. Let us be sure that in dealing with consumerism in the blindness field we not only try to get the right answers but also ask the right questions. Otherwise, we may lose an arm. (1990, pp. 102–106)

While describing exploitation and the custodial treatment which frequently characterizes employment in sheltered workshops, it is easy to lose sight of the individuals involved. In a letter to the *Braille Monitor,* a former blind employee of a sheltered workshop in Morristown, Tennessee, commented on the successful effort of the National Federation of the Blind to assist local workers in their efforts to organize for better work conditions and pay. He then reflects on his own experiences in the Morristown Workshop. I have included the introductory comments by the editor of the *Braille Monitor*.

LIFE AT THE MORRISTOWN WORKSHOP

Readers of the *Monitor* are familiar with the name of Edgar Sammons. He lives in the mountains of Tennessee, and his character and spirit are as rugged and individualistic as the hills he inhabits. From time to time Edgar writes me a letter.

He is not a world traveler, nor does he have an extensive academic education. Yet, he is an educated man. He is articulate and possessed of wisdom—wisdom which comes from a keen mind, a caring heart, a lifetime of experience, a lack of pretention, and the ability to cut through non-essentials to reality. I have always admired Edgar Sammons and regarded him as my friend.

His occasional letters help me keep things in perspective. They remind me of my heritage and background. They prevent me, as you might say, from getting above my raising.

Edgar formerly worked at the sheltered shop in Morristown. Recently he wrote me about it.

Mountain City, Tennessee

January 10, 1984

Here I am again. Thought I would try to write you a few lines as it is raining and I can't get out.

The blind won and won big in Morristown. I was glad to hear about it in the *Braille Monitor.* I hope it works. I worked there over sixteen and a half years. The workers who complained are right. The sighted people do a lot of work there that the blind could do. I don't remember now, but I think the shop moved to Morristown from Johnson City in 1956. I went down there and started training in 1956. They kept me on training for a year. They done that so the state would pay for it while the shop got the benefit of my work.

After I got off of training, I got seventy-five cents a hour. When I left there, I think I was getting a dollar and a half a hour. I beat the little felt beds for the army when they got orders for them. They got a good many orders for them the first few years that I worked there. I blowed and beat a lot of cotton mattresses. I covered springs and helped bag box springs and mattresses. They got a good many orders for mattress pads for a good while before I left there.

J.C. Austin put me to folding the pads and bagging and boxing them. I done just as much of that as the people that was getting full pay. I guess I was on that job for about two weeks. When I would catch up and get ahead, I would make a few cotton beds.

I went back to bag my pads one day, and a sighted woman said, "From now on I am bagging the beds, Edgar." I don't know whether J.C. Austin told her to do it or not. She bagged a while and turned it over to her sighted sister.

J.C. was floor boss at the time. I thought, "If he didn't tell her to take my job, why didn't he ask me why I wasn't bagging pads?" I didn't care. I wasn't getting any more pay anyway.

He might have thought that I had rather do something else. That wasn't the thing of it. The blind could do a lot more work in these shops if they had the training. They get the blind in there and get them on the welfare and just pay them a little. A blind person would have to get on the welfare with what they get paid. I went down there to work and try to get off of the welfare. They cut me down to eight dollars a month. I told them that I would have to come home if that was all I could get. They added a five dollar laundry allowance to my check. That let me make thirteen dollars a month. I was getting eighteen dollars a week on training period. I probably wouldn't have come home anyway because I didn't have anything else to do, and I needed something—something to let me do useful work even if I only got starvation pay.

One of the officials, Mrs. Goodman, said when I got off training she wanted to adjust my welfare check. She adjusted it all right. She adjusted it out and that was the last of that. They changed the law on it in a few years after Mattie Ruth and I got married. They tried to get us back on the welfare but we told them that we didn't want to. I don't think the foreman liked it.

I have been gone from there for over ten years. The one's that I knew when I was there didn't stick with the one's that did do something. I guess they was like me. I thought if we tried to do something, I might get laid off and have to go back and live off my people. While I was out on my own I meant to keep it that way. If the National Federation of the Blind had been there at the time, it might have made a lot of difference.

Mattie Ruth and I was married twenty-one years the 19th of November. If it was to do over, we would do it again. We have had a good bit of sickness, but we managed.

I have done a many of a hard day's work in that shop in Morristown, and they know it. I didn't get a raise the last year I worked there. They had stopped making cotton beds, but there were a lot of other things I could have done if they would have let me. Well, I hope the shop does right by the blind. A lot of people that they called blind had a lot of sight. There are very few that are totally blind. They ought to teach the blind a lot of things that they don't. (Jernigan, 1984c, pp. 84–86)

James Gashel is the staff member of the National Federation of the Blind assigned to work on legislation and governmental affairs. He has helped promote successful legislation in Congress and has worked on many cases involving the individual rights of blind people involving state and federal programs. He has had a major role in providing leadership and assistance to blind workers attempting to improve their position in sheltered workshops. Although the results described below are still not characteristic of sheltered workshops, it demonstrates what can be accomplished by the organized blind.

HOUSTON LIGHTHOUSE LABOR CONTRACT SIGNED FIRST IN NATION'S HISTORY

It's now official. Beginning September 4, 1983, all production and maintenance employees in Workshop A of the Lighthouse for the Blind of Houston are working under a labor agreement negotiated with the Lighthouse by the Teamsters Union Local No. 968. The agreement was ratified by the blind and sighted employees in the bargaining unit on September 1, 1983, and extends for a period of four years, through August 31, 1987. The official signing by Lighthouse and Union representatives occurred on September 22, 1983, putting an end to a legal battle which dates back nearly five years.

The history of the Houston struggle is a classic example of our increasing organizational effectiveness. It took a long time to achieve the final victory. The outcome was never certain. But we did not waiver in our commitment to see the battle through. Even when it appeared that we might lose—when the federal appeals court said, in August, 1981, that the National Labor Relations Act did not apply to the Lighthouse—we did not give up. We continued to use every appeal open to us. We pressed on. This is why one day the blind will be recognized for what we are, citizens who deserve equal treatment and first-class status.

Early in 1983, the same court that had previously ruled against the interests of the blind workers in Houston dramatically reversed itself and found that factory work, not rehabilitation, is the predominant enterprise of the Lighthouse. The Lighthouse of Houston had no hope for appeal. The new decision conformed to an earlier ruling by the Fifth Circuit Court of Appeals, giving workers at the Cincinnati Association for the Blind coverage under the National Labor Relations Act. The Supreme Court had declined to overturn the Cincinnati ruling and would certainly maintain the same posture in the Houston case, there being no disagreement between the circuits.

Reaching this point gobbled up years of litigation, not to mention much financial support provided by blind persons and their friends, nationwide. But the battle was not in vain. Collective bargaining was now a mandate, not a dream. The next step would be a labor agreement, or the Lighthouse would be subject to heavy penalties for refusing to bargain.

The agreement now in effect is a standard labor contract, covering virtually all aspects of the relationship between the Lighthouse and its production and maintenance workers (blind and sighted alike) in the bargaining unit. In all, there are some forty major provisions relating to wages, fringe benefits, days and hours of work, vacation days, sick leave, work rules, and grievance procedures—you name it. Just reading the contract, although it is a trifle tedious, is an education in itself. It is the first negotiated labor pact in the nation's history in a sheltered workshop, resulting from proceedings before the National Labor Relations Board and appeals in the federal courts.

This alone gives the contract historic significance. But the document is also a living instrument now to be used by blind shopworkers throughout the country. The very existence of this contract proves that the collective bargaining process will not destroy a sheltered workshop, despite what we have repeatedly been told by National Industries for the Blind and the people who run the workshops. And the result of collective bargaining need not be feared either, unless the bosses of the shops have something to hide. This, too, is proved by the contract. After all, the Lighthouse management in Houston agreed to all of the terms. The provisions of the agreement are responsible and balanced. They are fair to all parties. Such an agreement is by definition a meeting of the minds.

So, it is now on record that managers and workers in workshops can sit down at the bargaining table and hammer out an accord that everyone can live with. How can any workshop justifiably contend that this is wrong? Here are a few of the particulars: . . . (Omitted material includes the following topics—wages, pension plan, sick leave, vacations, holidays and holiday pay, pay guarantees and hours of work, disputes and grievances, bulletin boards and other provisions.) . . . So, there it is—our first labor contract in history covering a sheltered workshop. The management professionals said it *could* never be done, but we did it. NAC (the National Accreditation Council for Agencies Serving the Blind and Visually Handicapped) said it *should* never be done, but it happened all the same. It was ever thus with NAC, always on the wrong side of an issue and ever willing to fight against the blind. But against these forces, with all of their money and all of the power it can buy for them, we prevailed. We did not quit or lose our nerve. We did not sit back and let someone else take the heat. We were in the thick of the battle from the very beginning until the absolute end.

We have written another chapter in the struggle of the blind to rise up from second-class status and to be recognized as equals. Immediately the contract brought better wages and improved conditions to the blind at the Houston Lighthouse. It is estimated that in monetary terms this agreement alone will mean as much as $300,000 or more in increased pay and benefits during its four-year life.

But the ramifications of this single victory go far beyond the money which will now be paid to the blind workers in Houston who have actually earned it. The implications are enormous. Now with this agreement under our belts, shopworkers and the blind who march beside them everywhere in our country can look to the Houston pact and realize the possibilities that now exist. If we can win such an outstanding victory the first time out in Houston, why can't we do the same in Dallas, or in Chicago? Why can't we do it in Minneapolis or in

New York? Why not everywhere? It is only a matter of time. The Houston story is the story of our struggle of the blind to be free, and the contract which resulted from that struggle is now the promise of tomorrow. (Gashel 1984, pp. 24–28)

Chapter 8

EDUCATION AND REHABILITATION
FOR SELF-DETERMINATION

As the British sociologist, Bauman (1988), observed, "The competence of sociology ends where the future begins" (p. 89). While sociologists can provide information and ideas which enrich public debate and citizen discourse, they cannot provide the answers to social problems. They can help us consider the possible consequences of alternative social arrangements, and they can clarify underlying values of interest groups. In this sense, all social scientists are moral philosophers (Wolfe, 1989). Their research either supports present social arrangements or exposes those conditions which subordinate people without power and wealth.

Throughout this book, I have tried to explain the consequences for blind people who are continually kept in subordinate positions in social arrangements. I have focused on professions and agencies that dominate resources and social relationships in the rehabilitation and education of blind people. In Chapter 2, I analyzed the concept of human rights and how such values and ideals can be implemented through participation in the democratic process. Consumers become empowered when they organize themselves and mobilize human and economic resources to better pursue their goals. In the resulting social movements, new communities and subcultures develop.

> Sociologists find such developments interesting and important, as they may crack the magic circle of bureaucracy and consumer freedom by introducing a third, heretofore neglected, alternative: that of individual autonomy pursued through communal cooperation and grounded in communal self-rule. (Bauman, 1988, p. 95)

Freedom in the context of this type of community means the freedom to participate in terms of equality in the state and society. It does not mean isolation in the backwaters of the main stream. A first step toward this freedom to participate has been the redefinition of blindness itself for members of the community. This is a continuous process: each generation is challenged to reject internalized negative self images which have been learned from parents, peers, professionals, and people in the wider society. Positive images are affirmed and sustained in the activities of the social movement. In addition, as the organized blind challenge barriers to participation in society, professionals and the public become educated. The long white cane and Braille are the legacy of these challenges, both as symbols and tools of independence, and they are major elements in the subculture which has evolved. A cultural heritage and a sense of generational continuity has developed, and the only acceptable basis of interaction is in terms of equality, mutual respect and mutual regard. For the blind to be seen primarily as flawed vessels to be mended or as intrinsically different from other people is not acceptable.

How can this developing community most effectively incorporate its concerns into the education and rehabilitation process? This is the obvious starting point. If rehabilitation programs and agencies produce dependency rather than autonomy, how can more be expected from presumably less knowledgeable employers and citizens in the wider community? In the following pages, I will try to answer these questions, both in terms of ideals and social arrangements which would be most consistent with the aspirations of blind people for self-determination, autonomy, responsibility and equality of opportunity.

Desirable Organization or Agency Characteristics

Those who are employed to provide educational and rehabilitation services must have experience and ideas appropriate for teaching independence and self reliance. Many of these workers should be blind, not simply to give them employment, but to have qualified, competent, and broadly experienced blind people as role models for new clients and students. For rehabilitation agencies, having a significant number of blind employees can be a bonus. Teaching by example—successful role modeling—provides an invaluable introductory lesson to the student entering an educational or rehabilitation program.

However, nothing is worse than incompetent blind counselors and teachers. Judy Sanders, Minnesota office manager for Congressman Jerry Sikorski, described to me an instance involving a negative role model (personal communication, November 10, 1992). She had accompanied a prospective client to an initial meeting with a rehabilitation counselor who was continually apologetic because a reader was unexpectedly unavailable to him. For this reason, the counselor did not have the requisite documents ready. After spending an hour of the client's time, the counselor told her that they could make little progress that day and she would need to return another time. Regardless of the excuse, for the student this was an extremely poor example of professional competence. When blind or partially sighted employees are not self-reliant nor familiar with alternative techniques, it is a commentary on the level of performance acceptable to his or her agency. More than organizational inefficiency, examples of individual incompetence can greatly harm a person entering the rehabilitation process.

As I indicated in Chapter 2, agency employees should have had successful work experience before coming to an agency. Finding and maintaining competitive employment is better understood if one has experienced it him/herself. In addition, the worker will have a broader perspective on the variety of job aspirations held by clients. Reflecting on his work experience at the Iowa Commission for the Blind, James Omvig (1983) observed:

> If a blind person wished to join the staff, he or she must first successfully have held some other job in competitive employment to demonstrate both to that individual and to others that regular, competitive work is possible for the blind. Because of this experience, such a blind staff member would be in the best possible position to give real help and guidance. He or she could then serve as a role model for blind clients and would be much more credible to blind clients. (p. 88)

In addition, blind people should not be disproportionately restricted to entry level positions. Ability, when present, should be considered in opportunities for upward mobility. Like women employed in universities or women facing barriers to upper level positions in corporations, blind people are, but should not be, under-represented in administrative and management positions. This is not only a matter of fairness, but an additional component of successful rolemodeling. It is also a way of ensuring that appropriate philosophies about blindness are maintained in positions of power at higher levels in the agency.

Does this mean that people with normal vision have to be second class citizens in such work settings? Not at all. It does mean that the sighted person can no longer be king in the world of the blind. However, to be useful the sighted person must be "wise" (Goffman, 1961). She or he must have an empathic understanding of the array of problems confronted by blind people. Sleepshade training, a technique which simulates blindness for a sighted employee, can be used to sensitize workers to the conditions encountered by blind students. This is a requirement for employees at the Colorado Center for the Blind. In one instance, a teacher had been unable to teach a reluctant student how to light a gas oven. Consequently, the teacher told the student that she herself would use sleepshades and follow the directions for lighting the oven in order to see if she was leaving something out of the instructions. When sighted employees utilize sleepshades, it helps to give them confidence in what blind people can accomplish (D. McGeorge, Director of the Colorado Center for the Blind, personal communication, November 9, 1992). Many such techniques aid the teaching/learning process.

Beyond the usual education requirements, employees must have a positive philosophy about blindness. They should be willing to be involved in the social movement of the organized blind, an ongoing source of education for the professional. If by attitude or lack of appropriate knowledge, workers, regardless of the amount of vision they have, are barriers to autonomy and self reliance, they exploit both clients and supporters of the agency. They extract much, an occupation and a career, while contributing little. In fact, the net result of their efforts may be harmful and further propagate negative self-images and dependency.

The agency should involve representatives of the organized blind at all levels of decision making. They should be a significant presence at board meetings, on executive committees and on advisory boards. They should be recommended to the agency by the organized blind community in which they are known for their integrity, accomplishments and philosophy about blindness. Such representatives should be elected or otherwise formally selected from within the blindness community. For the agency to select outsiders is not acceptable.

Critics observe that most blind people do not belong to organizations of blind people, but that they also should be represented. However, such individuals represent no one but themselves. Their success rests upon token board memberships or agency positions for which they are selected because their ideas complement existing agency interests. (see also Chapter 2.)

> While you can always get an expression of the attitude you want through careful "selection," this practice has no place in the agency which has the best interests of the blind at heart. Such "individuals" have no reason to have any knowledge about what is needed. Meaningful information and input can be gathered only from those who have had the good sense to join together and to share ideas and experiences — the organized blind. (Omvig, 1983, p. 89)

This process averts the depoliticization of consumers that I described in Chapter 2. Tokenism at any level is not acceptable.

> The Agency, from the director on down, must be willing to "listen" to what the blind have to say and to work in a spirit of partnership with the organized blind. We are the persons affected by the services and we have a right to have a voice in what those services will be. Through our collective experience, we know well what works and what doesn't—what is good and what is bad. (p. 89)

The topic of representation is still a vital one as is reflected in a recent issue of the *Journal of Visual Impairment and Blindness,* September 1992, which focused on the blindness system. In consecutive annual Helen Keller Seminars sponsored by the American Foundation for the Blind, an array of committees considered various aspects of the blindness system. The committees included a consumer work group which discussed consumer interests. This group of ten included both sighted and blind, as well as several prominent people in the Association for the Rehabilitation and Education of the Blind and Visually Impaired (AER). However, none were active participants in the consumer movement which has consistently raised questions about the blindness system. Concerning representation, the report stated, "Simply put, consumers who belong to organizations for blind people may or may not represent the view of all blind people" (Wiener et al, 1992, p. 349). Such a statement presumes that anyone can represent blind people. The participants were encouraged to abandon their "stripes" and to "step out of traditional roles" (p. 349). Presumably, these professionals now represented consumers' interests.

Following the completion of this series of Helen Keller Seminars, the editor of the *Journal of Visual Impairment and Blindness* judged one evaluation response important enough to be included in her prologue to the issue on the state of the blindness system. Concerning consumer interests, Mulholland (1992) commented,

> At the last session of the 2nd year there was overwhelming consensus on one point: that the time when such a process could be done only with professionals was over. The tie that bound the system together was persons who are blind or visually impaired. (p. 314)

This conclusion has been maintained consistently by the National Federation of the Blind for more than fifty years, but is still resisted by many agencies and professionals who generally oppose representative consumer involvement.

Organizational Size

Bigger may not always be better when considering the delivery of rehabilitation and educational services. I have observed three rehabilitation agencies which, although independent, reflect the philosophy of the National Federation of the Blind. All are intentionally small in size and typically employ a staff of eight workers for sixteen to twenty resident students. Surprisingly, the monthly cost per student in such small agencies is frequently less than that in large rehabilitation centers.

BLIND (Blind Learning in New Dimensions), Inc., is located in Minneapolis. Five of its current seven board members are blind, since the agency's constitution requires that the majority of board members be so. All of the board members are currently active in organizations of blind people. According to Janet Lee, Vice-President of BLIND, Inc., having a blind administrator and staff members who have experienced competitive employment and have had positive experiences with their blindness are important considerations in staff recruitment.

Four of the present eight staff members are blind. In larger agencies, staff specialization and departmental separation may mean that the staff members themselves may not be well-acquainted. At BLIND, Inc., not only do the staff members know each other and work well as a team, they are also expected to become well acquainted with each student. According to the director, Joyce Scanlan, students, some of whom are still adolescents, are treated as adults who will rise to new responsibilities assigned in the training experience. Regarded as peers, they participate in social events with the staff from whom they learn social and other skills through frequent interaction. Staff members are committed to the progress of each student, and they work well beyond the eight hour day. "Students learn from each other's successes and each other's difficulties; this can only occur in a small group setting" (personal communication, September 26, 1992).

Scanlan observes that students coming to the program almost always have negative expectations of what blind people can do or accomplish. Critical to the program's success is that the students quickly and frequently interact with other blind people who are socially and economically successful. They soon develop confidence in the competence of the staff. Rather than only talking about independence, students observe and experience it through other students and staff.

At the Colorado Center for the Blind, the staff members involve themselves directly in teaching experiences intended to challenge student ideas about what is possible. For example, a required part of the curriculum is eight days of instruction in rock climbing. Using an existing business which teaches rock climbing to the general public, students are challenged to attempt and succeed in doing something they have never imagined possible. Heightened self-confidence is the result. Reluctant students are challenged by staff example and encouragement. A twelve year old boy who came to the Colorado Center with very little self-confidence and who expressed great reluctance to try rock climbing commented, "My favorite activity was going rock climbing. My favorite rock climbing instructor was Allison. The reason why I liked Allison so much was because she wouldn't let you come down the rock until you finished" (D. McGeorge, personal communication, November 8, 1992).

At BLIND, Inc., Scanlan observes that many students come to the program initially having more confidence in the sighted members of the staff. This quickly changes and bonding occurs. Negative opinions are not created about the sighted staff, but new levels of appreciation and respect develop concerning the qualities of the blind staff (personal communication, November 26, 1992). This often carries over into long term relationships as social networks develop. Students are challenged not only to develop positive self images, but to join in challenging others. The small size of the organization permits interaction in the homes of staff members and in diverse settings outside the normal curriculum. "As our students interact with blind members of the staff, whose lives have been successful as attorneys, teachers, social workers, counselors, and so forth, the negative images first projected by the blind students toward the blind staff simply cannot be maintained in face of the evidence" (J. Lee, personal communication, September 26, 1992).

The program is intentionally not associated with a sheltered workshop. This would necessarily increase organizational size and introduce patterns of dependency contrary to the aims of this organization. The philosophy is not to learn what one cannot do, but to build on what one can do. It is easy enough to learn what one cannot do on his or her own. This program encourages the staff to exhibit independent skills throughout the organization. I was told of an otherwise competent Braille teacher whom BLIND, Inc., would not employ because she was dependent on other staff members for message transmission rather than independently using alternative media. At the Colorado Center, staff members are expected to handle such problems themselves instead of exposing students to unnecessary examples of dependency.

Sometimes it is difficult—if not impossible—for staff members to express in their behavior their philosophy of independence. They may encounter resistance in larger agencies dominated by sighted or blind individuals with traditional philosophies about custodial care. The effort of a teacher to become more effective and a positive role model can become a threat in the traditional agency. In fact, Scanlan has observed that workers in larger centers are sometimes rewarded for their willingness to be dependent upon other staff members. They are rewarded for being led around rather than for traveling independently because the former maintains the status quo. Also, in larger public agencies there is the additional problem of the accumulation of minimally competent people because it is difficult to remove them. Learning from such teachers, who often appear to have little confidence in other blind people, is one of the most deadening experiences a student can encounter. Staff members who demonstrate unnecessary dependency or anything less than the highest levels of accomplishment are not acceptable in small agencies where each person is critical.

Traditional credentials, such as a master's degree in orientation and mobility, are not necessary in this program (Dodds, 1986). A prospective staff member needs to demonstrate competence in other ways. Many argue that much of what professionals learn in graduate degree programs is contrary to autonomous living. Such people, whether blind or not, may not have experienced competitive employment outside the agency. As I noted in Chapter 2, this may result in narrowed expectations.

The Agency as Advocate

An agency should be a strong advocate for the rights of blind people and it should make efforts to educate the public. Its allegiance should be to consumers and to other agencies which operate under a philosophy that leads to independent living and self-determination for blind people. If the agency is viewed as paternalistic or custodial by its prospective clients, its programs will surely be less effective. "The good agency must be an 'advocate' for the civil rights of all blind persons. It must be willing to become involved and to have confrontations. However, it must be mindful of the fact that it does not 'represent' anybody. Only those elected by others can do that" (Omvig, 1983, p. 89). This is true not only for the agency in the local community, but for agencies and organizations which designate themselves nationwide authorities.

Throughout its fifty years, the National Federation of the Blind has insisted that it is an organization *of* the blind. I have frequently heard professionals in leadership positions claim that the distinction between designations such as "of the blind" and "for the blind" is unimportant or trivial. However, when agencies insist that they are agencies *for* the blind, they reveal that they do not adequately comprehend issues of consumer participation or the empowerment of blind people in matters that involve them. If agencies and the organized blind community become partners, their combined human and economic assets will result in a more effective use of resources and almost certainly in better education and rehabilitation services.

Physical Setting

An effective rehabilitation process requires a good orientation center. This is the place where students learn travel, communication and independent living skills. There they learn to be reflective about their potential and the best way to reach their goals. Accordingly, the setting should not be an isolated campus where services are self-contained. Conditions for living and learning should be similar to those that will be encountered in the wider community. For example, one large, well known center for training blind people has sheltered walkways leading from the dormitory and the administration building and special railings for guidance purposes. The cafeteria has raised carpet walkways. Instead of learning to serve themselves, students hold up a hand and the number of fingers they display indicates their beverage choice. Obviously, such arrangements do not produce independence either in the orientation center or life outside it.

As indicated in Chapter 5, environmental "safety" devices are usually not warranted. Textured subway platforms, beeping mass transit doors, and ringing bells at street crossings are unnecessary and wasteful of public money. As reflected in the consumer literature, they are often more dangerous because they add to existing levels of noise, are not present at all locations, and do not provide information that a well-trained blind traveler can not obtain by ordinary means. For example, the ringing bell that indicates that a traffic light has changed from green to red does not indicate whether a driver has obeyed the law. The properly trained blind traveler is far safer when she or he has determined that traffic has stopped.

In addition to their cost and near uselessness as safety devices, most of these environmental adaptations heighten public stereotypes of blind people. They suggest that blind people require major public intervention for their own safety. For similar reasons, special access offices for blind students receiving higher education are both unnecessary and harmful. Almost every university has them (see Chapter 2). At my university a staff member from the access office contacts me to tell me that a blind person is in my class. Prior to each examination I am called by a member of that staff who arranges to pick up the exam, give it to the student, and then return it to me. Why should the student not learn to do this by himself or herself? As an instructor, I regret the lost opportunity of interacting with these students. Not only are such programs expensive, they further the isolation of blind students, encourage their dependency on "special arrangements," and reduce opportunities for them to be responsible for their own lives.

In the Main Stream

A great majority of blind children now attend non-residential schools. The traditional schools for the blind, in general, have fewer students and they are usually multiply handicapped. Children whose only impediment to learning is blindness are increasingly likely to attend regular schools.

The quality of the education received by these children is a growing concern among the parents of blind children and the blindness community in general. The advantages of mainstreaming will avail little if blind children do not receive the basic tools to enable them to learn effectively. If Braille, mobility instruction, and proper philosophy about blindness are not effectively taught, the student will not be successful in either the sighted or blind community. Her or his communication skills, and thus autonomy, will be greatly limited. Teachers with only a general special education background may not have the requisite knowledge necessary to educate blind students for competitive employment and independent living. Students must have competent teachers if they are to learn the alternative techniques available for autonomy and self-reliance. If the student later chooses alternatives other than Braille, no harm has been done (Ianuzzi, 1992; Schroeder, 1992). If the student learns it well, he or she will have a choice and one of those choices will always include self-reliance (Eckery, 1991).

Accountability

As I described in Chapter 7, accountability is at the heart of agency controversy. The National Accreditation Council for Agencies Serving the Blind and Visually Handicapped focuses, for example, on physical facilities and formal staff qualifications (see Chapter 6). However, evaluation should focus on outcome, not only to avoid wasting scarce resources, but also to assure results consistent with the goals of rehabilitation. In the short view this means determining whether or not students have learned valued skills and attitudes. In the longer view, it refers to the consequences the required skills and attitudes have for vocational success and independent living. For example, BLIND, Inc., in its annual report for 1991, listed the outcome of its rehabilitation efforts.

> Twenty-six students participated in the comprehensive training program in 1991. Of those, three remain in training. Those who have left the program are doing the following:
>
>   10—attending high school or college
>   6—employed
>   4—seeking employment
>   3—living independently
>
> (BLIND, Inc., 1991, pp. 2–3)

Whatever else the future holds for these individuals, the report suggests that they have not become dependent on the agency and are living independently and continuing their education and employment.

Accountability, program evaluation and policy analysis are almost always included in requests for funding from governmental resources or private foundations. Frequently, data is collected but not analyzed. It is often easy to acquire and impute on a computer format. However, in the absence of special funding for evaluative research, staff members with the time and competence for data analysis are not available. Frequently, the data obtained is of little use; it is too narrow in its focus or simply useless for assessing the value of programs. At other times it may be judged politically sensitive and thus not utilized.

In order to illustrate several dimensions of this discussion, I will describe a few aspects of a recent program evaluation effort in Minnesota. The Department of Jobs and Training, State Services for the Blind currently contracts with three private agencies in Minnesota to provide alternative techniques for blind people to pursue their vocational and rehabilitation interests more efficiently. These are the Duluth Lighthouse for the Blind, the Minneapolis Society for the Blind, and the afore mentioned Blind: Learning in New Dimensions (BLIND, Inc.).

> Perhaps the most difficult goal a government agency can undertake is measuring the effectiveness of its services. To its credit, SSB [Minnesota State Services for the Blind] undertook such a goal in May and June, 1990. The measurement consisted of a survey of its clients and staff. (National Federation of the Blind of Minnesota, Inc., n.d.)

During the months following the collection of the data, the resulting information was, to some degree, analyzed. This became known when the director of Minnesota State Services for the Blind, Mr. Rick Hokanson, mentioned in a presentation to the National Federation of the Blind of Minnesota that some differences had emerged concerning the effectiveness of the three agencies. BLIND, Inc., is closely associated in both philosophy and staffing with the National Federation of the Blind of Minnesota. The leadership of this agency thought BLIND, Inc., to be the most effective. The National Federation of the Blind wanted to know more about the evaluation survey.

As discussed in Chapters 2 and 3, citizen requests such as this can be awkward for agency administrators. First, the state agency must protect the confidentiality of the clients interviewed. Second, the politics of spending public money is involved. There is a tendency to provide continuing support for established agencies because they are visible within their communities and represent community economic resources. To eliminate or greatly reduce such contracts might greatly jeopardize agencies and careers. In every state, long term agency personnel establish many professional ties with long term agency staff members working in parallel state bureaucracies: they have common interests and it is good for business. For these reasons, and perhaps others, the data has not been made public. Or, to judge by subsequent contract allocations, the policy implications had not been taken seriously.

For whatever reason, cooperation from the State Services for the Blind was not judged adequate. "To resolve these conflicting statements and see what the results really were, the National Federation of the Blind of Minnesota requested the survey forms under the Minnesota Government Data Practices Act" (T. Scanlan, 1992). After properly assuring client anonymity, the Minnesota State Services for the Blind released the raw data. The NFB of Minnesota, a volunteer consumer organization, analyzed the data and focused on the program outcome of each agency. "The measure of training effectiveness [was] the use of skills after leaving the facility" (National Federation of the Blind of Minnesota, Inc., n.d., p. 1). From the point of view of the NFB of Minnesota,

> The findings of [the] survey confirm the wisdom of the 1991 Legislature in amending state law (MSA Chapter 248.07). That amendment instructs the Department of Jobs and Training to increase the use of consumer-controlled training facilities which emphasize skills such as Braille and white-cane use and develop positive attitudes. (p. 3)

The following charts were based on data collected by the staff for the Minnesota State Services for the Blind. With regard to the question concerning what students did with their lives after leaving the training facilities, the first shows that the difference in the outcomes for those involved in the three agencies was great.

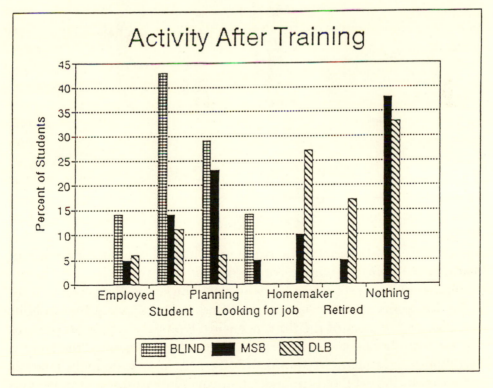

(National Federation of the Blind of Minnesota, n.d., p.6)

Concerning the use of Braille, BLIND, Inc., reported more than twice the percentage of students using it every week. More than 55 percent from BLIND, Inc., reported weekly use, while only 12 percent from the Duluth Lighthouse for the Blind did so. Activities for daily living included grooming, upkeep of clothing, cooking, housekeeping, sewing, shopping, and so forth. Similarly, for these tasks there were pronounced differences between the agencies.

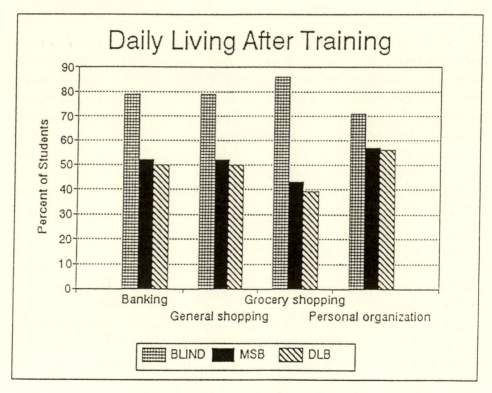

(National Federation of the Blind of Minnesota, n.d., p.9)

The Duluth Lighthouse for the Blind was the weakest on all measures of the NFB of Minnesota analysis of the data.

Another dimension to this survey involved questions directed to the staff of the Minnesota State Services for the Blind. The staff was asked about its attitudes toward each of the three agencies. Ironically, the most positive staff feelings about agency performance were directed toward the Duluth Lighthouse and the lowest toward BLIND, Inc. According to the analysis conducted by the NFB of Minnesota, there are clear differences in the performances of these agencies when the outcome for clients is the measure.

The counselors feel the most positive about the less effective training programs. As much as they may deny it, these feelings will affect their counseling of their clients. The result (intended or not) will be to steer the blind clients toward less effective training and less independent lives. (p. 14)

The sequence of events surrounding the Minnesota State Services for the Blind's program evaluation efforts can be viewed many ways; first, since the Minnesota SSB of is a state agency, usually regarded as progressive, collected data concerning agency performance was being paid for by taxpayers through federal and state revenues. At some future time, the data would have been used for policy analysis and staff training and attention would have been given to the most effective use of public money. Two, because of the politics involved in spending public money and giving contracts to sustain established agencies, little would have been done with this data. Not only would there have been political pressure from outside the state agency, there would have been political pressure from within. This would have come from long-term staff members with professional and, sometimes, social ties to the more established agencies. Even the most dedicated leadership would have had difficulty dealing with the data objectively. Progress, if any, is usually slow.

Three, these events can be viewed as squabbling between three agencies continually seeking to expand their economic resources. It is important, perhaps even critical to their programs that they receive contracts. An agency can be financially destroyed if counselors direct students elsewhere. Even with the freedom of choice concerning pilot projects being included in the reauthorization of the Vocational Rehabilitation Act of 1992, counselors have much influence over newly blind clients or clients isolated from consumer organizations.

Four, the analysis indicates that public money is not being well spent. According to the NFB of Minnesota, BLIND, Inc., with which they are closely associated, clearly provides programs resulting in greater self-confidence, independent living, and employment—as indicated from the data collected by the State of Minnesota itself. The group is equally concerned about the other two agencies, not only because scarce resources are wasted, but because blind people are being harmed by poor education and training practices. These agencies are considered barriers rather than doorways to full community participation.

This accountability incident illustrates the integrity of this particular consumer organization and the dedication of its membership. Volunteers spent much time and money analyzing data collected by the state agency. The individuals involved got no pleasure from the conflict which resulted from the efforts to obtain information. However the reader views these events, I pay careful attention to the stated goals and ideas of thoughtful citizens demonstrating concern about programs using public money and possibly having negative consequences for clients. Empowerment means many different things including representative participation on decision making boards, taking the initiative to generate information, and influencing present and future policy decisions. The challenge is to keep the consumer movement vital as it grows in organizational size, complexity, and resources. It will need to find ways to continually renew its commitment to its goals.

Ideas About Blindness

As I have often repeated, the only significant difference between the blind and others is the amount of vision, and with proper education and training this one difference can be reduced to little more than a nuisance. Employees of a successful agency will have positive outlooks about blindness and they will be enthusiastic supporters of and participants in the organized blind movement and take some pride in the contribution that many educators and counselors have made to this movement. The energy and commitment of blind people themselves to improving the lives of others is a remarkable contribution to rehabilitation efforts. Using their own resources and acting upon ideals of democracy and human rights, they are, despite much opposition, redefining what it means to be blind.

In this book I have described many sources of conflict. One attracting intense interest in the blind community in recent years is the increasing rate of illiteracy among blind people. This issue reached the front page of the *New York Times* in 1991. From 1965 to 1989 the literacy rate for visually handicapped students dropped from 50 percent to 12 percent (DeWitt, 1991). The argument over Braille concerns who should learn it, who should make the decision, and the competency of teachers. The following article by the current president of the National Federation of the Blind, Marc Maurer (1991), appeared in the *Braille Monitor*. It reflects the position that most strongly promotes Braille literacy.

WHO SHOULD LEARN BRAILLE AND WHY?

Braille is the raised dot system used by the blind for reading and writing. Recent publicity about Braille has brought both information and confusion to the public.

As a blind person myself and as president of the nation's largest organization primarily composed of blind persons (the 50,000-member National Federation of the Blind), I think I know something about the needs of blind persons. A controversy now exists as to who should learn Braille and under what circumstances, but certain things are generally agreed upon. Blind children (and also adults) should make full use of computers, tape recorders, and any other available technology. Visually impaired children should be encouraged to make the best use of any eyesight they have, including learning to read print.

But a legally blind child (one with less than ten percent of normal eyesight) cannot function efficiently using print alone. Sighted children have computers and recorders, but they still learn to read print. They use both eyes and ears to get information. Likewise, if a blind or severely visually impaired child is to compete, not only ears but also fingers should be used. Technology enhances but does not substitute for the printed word.

Then why the controversy? Many of today's teachers of blind children take a single college course on how to teach Braille but cannot read or write it. Because of their lack of knowledge, they tend to think Braille is slow and inefficient. Being uncomfortable with what they don't know, they say that Braille is not needed and opt for expensive technology.

There is also the fact that blindness still carries with it a stigma, and many (including some parents and teachers) want blind children to pretend to have sight they don't possess so as not to be considered blind—the same thing blacks did fifty years ago when some tried to lighten their skins and straighten their hair to try to cross the color line. It didn't work and wasn't healthy for the blacks. The same is true for the blind. The National Federation of the Blind believes it is respectable to be blind, and we don't try to hide it.

Thousands of blind people read Braille at four hundred words per minute. There's no substitute for Braille in taking notes, reading a speech, looking up words in a directory, studying a complicated text, or just having the fun of reading for yourself. Talk of forcing blind children to learn Braille shows the prejudice. Nobody talks of forcing sighted children to learn print. It is taken for granted as a right, a necessary part of education; so it should be with Braille and blind children.

The National Federation of the Blind is asking state legislatures to pass Braille bills, which would require teachers of the blind and visually handicapped to be available to every visually handicapped child if parents want it. The National Federation of the Blind believes that no child is hurt by learning Braille, print, or any other skill. The federal act often cited as the excuse for not making Braille universally available to the blind is misquoted. The requirement that each child's individual needs be met was never meant as a cop-out for teachers and an excuse for illiteracy. Just as with the sighted, we the blind need every skill we can get to compete in today's world. With proper training we can hold our own with the best. (pp. 360–361)

Traditional ideas about blindness are continually being challenged by the organized blind movement. Changing what it means to be blind is a recurring theme, and each new generation of blind people and each newly blinded individual must participate. In terms of organizational leadership and published material, no one has contributed more in this area than Kenneth Jernigan (1970). The following speech reflects these goals and commitments.

BLINDNESS—THE MYTH AND IMAGE

It is not only individual human beings who suffer from what the psychologists call an "identity crisis"—that is, a confusion and doubt as to who and what they are. So do groups of human beings—communities, associations, minorities, even whole nations. And so it is—in this year of space if not of grace—with the blind, organized and unorganized. We are, as I believe, in the midst of our own full-fledged identity crisis. For the first time in centuries—perhaps in a millennium—our collective identity is in question. For the first time in modern history there are anguish and argument, not only as to what we are, but as to what we may become. The traditional images and myths of blindness, which had been taken for granted and for gospel throughout the ages, both by the seeing and by the blind themselves, are now abruptly and astonishingly under attack.

Who is it that dares thus to disturb the peace and upset the applecart of traditional definitions? The aggressors are here in this room. They are you and I. They are the organized blind of the National Federation. It is we who have brought on our own identity crisis—by renouncing and repudiating our old mistaken identity as the "helpless blind." It is we who are demanding that we be called by our rightful and true names: names such as *competent, normal,* and *equal.* We do not object to being known as *blind,* for that is what we are. What we protest is that we are not also known as *people,* for we are that, too. What we ask of society is not a change of heart (our road to shelter has always been paved with good intentions), but a change of *image*—an exchange of old myths for new perspectives.

Of all the roadblocks in the path of the blind today, one rises up more formidably and threateningly than all others. It is the invisible barrier of ingrained social attitudes toward blindness and the blind— attitudes based on suspicion and superstition, on ignorance and error, which continue to hold sway in men's minds and to keep the blind in bondage.

But new attitudes about the blind have come into being. They exist side by side with the old and compete with them for public acceptance and belief. Between the two there is vast distance and no quarter. As an example consider the following quotation: "The real problem of blindness is not the loss of eyesight. The real problem is the misunderstanding and lack of information which exist. If a blind person has proper training and if he has opportunity, blindness is only a physical nuisance" (Iowa Commission for the Blind, n.d.).

That is a quotation from an administrator in the field of work with the blind. Here is another quotation from another official: "We must not perpetuate the myth that blindness is not a tragedy. For each person who has learned to live an active, fruitful life despite blindness, there are thousands whose lives have lost all meaning ... A blind person can't be rehabilitated as a crippled person may be. You can give a [crippled] man mobility, but there is no substitute for sight" (Stein, 1967, p. 19).

Those two quotations represent the considered judgments of two professionals in the field of services to the blind. The statements are squarely contradictory. If one of them is true, the other must be false. Which are we to believe? There is no doubt as to which of the two would win a public opinion poll. The more popular by far is the second—the one that repudiates as a shocking fiction the very idea that blindness is anything less than a total tragedy.

Let us take note in passing of the peculiar tone of finality and conviction in which this second statement—the "hard line" on blindness—is expressed. I believe there is a striking irony in it which all of us would do well to recognize, for it conveys the distinct impression that there is something cruel and unfair to blind people in the mere-nuisance concept of blindness, as opposed to the evidently kinder and fairer portrayal of the condition as an overwhelming disaster.

The difference between these two perspectives on blindness is not merely that one is optimistic and the other pessimistic. There is more to it than that. The crucial difference is that one view minimizes the consequences of the physical disability and actively rejects the notion that blind persons are somehow "different." Its emphasis is upon the normality of the blind, their similarity and common identity with others, their potential equality, and their right to free and full participation in all the regular pursuits and pastimes of their society. The accent here, in a word, is *affirmative:* it is upbeat, dynamic, rehabilitative. It makes much of opportunity and capacity and does not dwell on deprivation and disability.

By contrast the other point of view—which we might call the "disaster" concept—deliberately maximizes the effects of blindness: physically, psychologically, emotionally, and socially. Its emphasis is upon what is missing rather than what can be done—upon lacks and losses rather than upon capacities and strengths. Blindness, these spokesmen are inclined to tell us, is a kind of "dying;" and those who are blind (so we are repeatedly informed) are *abnormal*—they are *different*—they are *dependent*—they are *deprived*—they are *inferior*—and above all, they are *unfortunate.* The accent here, in a word, is *negative.* It is downbeat, pessimistic; professionally condescending, frequently sanctimonious, and ultimately defeatist.

I submit that this disaster concept of blindness is not only a popular opinion among professionals and the public today. It is, with only a little updating and streamlining, the ancient myth of blindness—the classic image of the blind man as a *tragic figure.* Let me be clear about this use of the term *"tragic."* In its classical sense, tragedy is not mere unhappiness. It does not refer to accidental misfortune or limited harm, which can sensibly be overcome. Tragedy involves a sentence of doom, a dire destiny, which one can only confront in all its unalterable terror but can never hope to transcend. The sense of tragedy, in short, is the sense of calamity—to which the only appropriate response is resignation and despair. These words of Bertrand Russell convey the mood exactly: "On such a firm foundation of unyielding despair must the soul's habitation henceforth securely be built." (pp. 117–119)

After giving many examples of frivolous and dependency creating gadgetry being marketed for blind people, Dr. Jernigan introduces a quotation which Philip S. Platt presented to a group of professional workers.

To dance and sing, to play and act, to swim, bowl and roller-skate, to work creatively in clay, wood, aluminum or tin, to make dresses, to join in group readings or discussions, to have entertainments and parties, to engage in many other activities of one's own choosing—this is to fill the life of anyone with the things that make life worth living.

Let me remind you of the way in which Dr. Jacobus tenBroek, then in his prime as president of the National Federation of the Blind, responded to that statement. In one of his great convention speeches, "Within the Grace of God," he quoted the passage and went on to say this:

Are these the things that make life worth living for you? Only the benevolent keeper of an asylum could make this remark—only a person who views blindness as a tragedy which can be somewhat mitigated by little touches of kindness and service to help pass the idle hours but which cannot be overcome. Some of these things may be suitable accessories to a life well filled with other things—a home, a job, and the rights and responsibilities of citizenship, for example.

The point I am seeking to make now is the very same point that Dr. tenBroek was seeking to make then. There are two opposing conceptions of the nature of blindness at large in the world. One of them holds that it is a nuisance, and the other that it is a disaster. I think it is clear that the disaster concept is widespread alike in popular culture and in the learned culture of the professionals. Moreover, I would submit that the concept itself is the *real* disaster—the only real disaster that we as blind people have to live with—and that when we can overcome this monstrous misconception, we shall ring down the curtain forever on the fictional drama entitled "The Tragedy of Blindness."

In order to emphasize still further the full extent to which the disaster concept—the tragic sense of blindness—prevails among the professionals in our fields, let me introduce in evidence another exhibit. It is a comment from overseas by an official of the National Council for the Blind of Ireland. This is what he says of the blind people of his country:

Although the exceptional and stubborn can learn a trade or pursue an education up to university level [note that "up to"] *and follow successful careers, such cases are unusual. Since unemployment has always been a factor in our economy, there are not many posts available. We lack the industries with the necessary repetitive machinery on which the blind can safely work.*

All that needs to be remarked about that dreary pronouncement is that it heavily reinforces the defeatist notion that blind persons in general (those who are not peculiarly stubborn and exceptional) should give up any idea of pursuing a normal trade or even of attaining an ordinary education, and should resign themselves to the prospect (itself not too likely) that society in its kindness may be willing to set aside enough repetitive and mechanical chores to take care of most of them, in penury and penitence. . . . The blind people of yesterday, and the day before yesterday, had little choice but to accept the tragic view of the gloom-and-doom mongers—the prophets of despair. Their horizons were limited to the bounty of charity, and their world was bounded by the sheltered workhouse. At every turn they were reminded of their infirmity; on every occasion they were coaxed into immobility and dependency. It is no wonder that they fulfilled the prophecy of despair; believing it themselves, they made it come true.

But that was another time, another era, another world. We the blind people of today have carried out a revolution, and have won our independence. We have won it by finding our own voice, finding our own direction—and finding our own doctrine. That doctrine may be simply stated: it is that the blind are normal people who can not see. It is that blindness is not a dying—but a challenge to make a new life. It is also that there are none so blind as those who will not see this simple truth.

The blind people of today, in a word, were not born yesterday. We who are blind do not accept the tragic prophecies of a dire fate. We have a rendezvous with a different destiny. The destiny we go to meet is that of integration and equality—of high achievement and full participation—of free movement and unrestricted opportunity in a friendly land which is already beginning to accept us for what we are.

That is where the blind are leading the blind. Let those who would resist or deny that destiny remain behind, imprisoned in their own antique myths and images—while the rest of us move on to new adventure and higher ground. (pp. 122–125)

What the goals and ideals mean in the lives of ordinary people is the most important outcome of this consumer movement. Freedom includes both rights and responsibilities. It means the opportunity for a home, a job and to do as much with their lives as their energy, talent, and ambition permit. We always receive help from other people. Joanne Wilson is the director for the Louisiana Center for the Blind. Before she initiated a new rehabilitation center in Louisiana, she had been a successful student, wife, mother, and school teacher. "The Freedom Bell" is one of her recent speeches.

THE FREEDOM BELL

The Louisiana Center for the Blind gives to each of its students at their graduation party a plaque, and on the bottom of that plaque it says, "Together We Are Changing What it Means to be Blind." All of our students know that "together" means the National Federation of the Blind. It means what has been done since 1940. It means the beliefs, the goals, and the dreams of all of us. They know when they are in the Center, that it's not just the staff, and it's not just the other students or the former students or the Louisiana chapter. They know that it is the entire National Federation of the Blind. They know that what they accomplish is in our hopes, our beliefs, and our dreams. When they leave the Louisiana Center for the Blind, they know that there is a whole structure behind them in the form of the National Federation of the Blind. And most importantly, they know that they must give back to that structure. They must give back to the National Federation of the Blind and pass on the dreams and the beliefs and the opportunities that they have received at the Louisiana Center for the Blind.

The Louisiana Center for the Blind was started on October 1, 1985. We now own our own classroom building and our own apartment complex, which the students live in. We have students now coming to us not only from Louisiana but from seven other states.

We teach cane travel, typing, Braille, home economics—the usual courses that are taught in rehabilitation centers. But beyond all that, we teach genuine belief and hope and high expectations and confidence to our students. We teach them that they truly can change what it means to be blind.

One of the traditions that we have at Louisiana Center for the Blind is our freedom bell. We have a big old school bell (a hand-rung school bell) that sits up in our Braille room. Throughout our short history, whenever a student calls us with some success or some good news, when something very important happens that affects all of us as blind people, we ring the freedom bell. In the past few months we have rung the bell for George, who called up and said, "I got my first check today from the naval base." We rang the bell when Maria said, "I'm twenty-two years old, but this is the first time I went out and bought a dress for myself."

We rang the bell when John, our young lawyer, came running in. He had graduated from the program: "I haven't called my parents yet. I haven't told my girlfriend yet. I am telling you first. I just got a job as a lawyer."

We rang the bell after two trips down to the state legislature to work on the Braille law. We rang the bell when we found that the Braille law indeed got passed. We rang the bell for Lillian, who received her high school graduation equivalency diploma, and for the many other students who received their diplomas. We rang the bell when Nancy and John, two of our former students, got married. We rang the bell when Lina and Jimmy had their first baby. We rang the bell for our first play on opening night. We rang our bell when the first crop came in from our garden, when we had our first produce as blind people from our very own garden. We rang the bell when all of our nervous and scared students got back from Mardi Gras, an event that they had been dreading for weeks. They got through the crowds. They got through the mobs and proved to themselves inside that they could be successful, capable individuals.

We rang the bell when Maria was able to cross Bonner Street, a street which she was scared to death to cross with a cane. We ring the bell when our college students call in and say, "Hey, I passed a course, and I got a 3.0 average this semester."

We rang the bell when Patty passed her bar exam. She is now working as a public defender in Shreveport. We rang the bell when Barry began managing three restaurants in Shreveport, when S.J. got his vending stand, when Joie got his factory job working for Boeing Aircraft, when Connie got a job as a nurse, and when Yvonda successfully finished business school.

We rang the bell when our students successfully prepared and served a meal for forty. We are about ready to ring it again. One of our students is ready to go back to being an elementary school teacher and another back to being a scientist at Los Alamos National Laboratories in New Mexico. We have another student, who is about ready to graduate and go into child care.

We ring the bell when our students call up and say, "Hey, I was elected president of our local chapter, or vice president," or "I just joined my local chapter." We rang the bell when Zach and Sheena said, "We got Pennsylvania and New Jersey to send us to you. We want good rehabilitation training." We rang the bell when Chris lit her first fire on a camping trip.

These are all times when we rang the freedom bell, but the real truth is what happens to our students. Here, in their own words, is what a few of them have to say.

Zach Shore: My first day at the Center I went into cooking class, and I asked my instructor, "What should I make today?"

She said, "You are going to bake Andrea's birthday cake today." I thought she was insane. I'd never done that before, but she said, "You can do it." It really turned out to be pretty good.

When I got to my cane travel class on my second day, my instructor said, "Zach, I'm sending you out on a route today." He had me on the street on the second day, and a wave of panic came over me. This teacher is obviously a raving lunatic. I didn't think I could do it, but I did. I came back safely, and my travel is getting better. The staff is very good. They really care about us. They really push us to do what we don't think we can do, and we find that we really can.

Tom Ley: I'm currently a senior at Louisiana Tech, majoring in mathematics and physics education. Before attending the Center I had limited myself, simply because I didn't have confidence in myself as a blind person if it involved going into an unfamiliar situation or doing unfamiliar things. After being there for only a month and a half, I could feel the limiting bonds I had placed upon myself melting away, and my horizons expanding about me. That's a gift I can never repay except by working as hard as I can for the Federation and its goals.

Roland Allen: I completed my training at the Center about a year ago. When I left, I felt that I gained several important things. But the most important thing that I got from the Center was the fact that I have accepted my blindness. When I first went to the Center, I had planned on going to college, and I was real scared to go. I knew that I wouldn't make it with the skills I had. After I left the Center, I felt confident that I could get in there and do what I wanted to.

Cheryl Domingue: I, too, like Zach, when I first arrived at the Center, thought that not only was the cooking instructor insane, but that they all were insane having me do the things they wanted me to do. The thing I thought was more horrifying than anything else was having a blind travel instructor. I thought that was really crazy. But after a few days of being there, and after seeing what all of the other students who had been there for some time had done with themselves, and after I saw how well my blind instructors were doing, I figured if they could do it, so could I. I didn't have any confidence in myself at all when I came to the Center but now have all the confidence in the world in myself. I am now a college student. I completed my first semester at the Nickel State University with a 3.0 average. Without the support of my family and all the friends I have made in the National Federation of the Blind, and especially my two children (Sheila and Shawn) who are here with me, I could not have made it.

So there you have it. Let the freedom bell ring! (1992, pp. 33–43)

BIBLIOGRAPHY

Abbott, A. (1988). *The system of professions.* Chicago: University of Chicago Press.

Adam, B. (1978). *The survival of domination: Inferiorization in everyday life.* Elsevier, NY: Elsevier North Holland.

Ahrne, G. (1990). *Agency and organization: Towards an organizational theory of society.* New Park, CA: Sage.

Albrecht, G. L. and Levy, J. A. (1981). Constructing disabilities as social problems. In G. Albrecht (Ed.), *Cross national rehabilitation policies,* (pp. 11–32). Beverly Hills and London: Sage.

——. (1984). A sociological perspective of physical disability. In J. L. Ruffini (Ed.), *Advances in medical social science,* (Vol. 2). New York: Gordon and Breach.

Albrecht, G. (1992). *The disability business: Rehabilitation in America.* Walnut Creek, CA: Sage.

Altman, B. M. (1981). Studies of attitudes toward the handicapped: The need for a new direction. *Social Problems, 28,* 3.

American Association of Workers for the Blind (AAWB) *Proceedings.* (1935). Committee report.

Anonymous A. (1965, February). COMSTAC on agency function and structure. *Braille Monitor,* 1–5.

Anonymous B. (1966, February). COMSTAC—standards for physical facilities. *Braille Monitor,* 27–31.

Anonymous C. (1966, February). COMSTAC—stumbling blocks to independent travel for the blind. *Braille Monitor,* 52–60.

Arato, A., & Cohen, J. (1992). Civil society and social theory. In P. Beilharz and G. Robinson (Eds.), *Between totalitarianism and postmodernity* (pp. 199–219). Cambridge, MA: MIT Press.

Ashton, P. C. (1979). Rehabilitation in a major corporate setting. *Journal of Rehabilitation, 45* (3), 26–29.

Bauman, Z. *Freedom.* (1988). Minneapolis: University of Minnesota Press.

Best, H. (1934). *Blindness and the blind in the United States.* New York: Macmillan.

——. (1939). The need for standards in work for the blind. *Proceedings of the 18th Biennial Convention of the American Association of Workers for the Blind, 33* (20).

BLIND, Inc. (1991). *Annual Report.* Minneapolis, MN.

Bogdan, R., et al. (1982, Fall). The disabled: Media's monster. *Social Policy,* 32–35.

Bolte, B. (1992). Jerry's kidding. *In These Times, 16,* (36–37), 24.

Brandy, K. (1991, October). Group pickets benefit for the blind. *Braille Monitor,* 572–574.

Brown, C. (1988, May/June). The Richmond workshop: Bad management, "quality services," and NAC. *Braille Monitor,* 228–230.

Burkhardt, P. (1984, September). A question of custodialism. *Braille Monitor,* 426–428.

Cahill, J. I. (1976). *Summary and critique of available data on the prevalence and economic and social costs of visual disorders and disabilities.* Prepared for the U.S. Department of Health and Welfare Public Health Service. Rockville, MD: Westate. (Available from the American Foundation of the Blind.)

Carney, N. (1992, November). The Federal Rehabilitation Act: Now and in the future. *Braille Monitor,* 590–593.

Carroll, T. J. (1961). *Blindness: what it is, what it does, and how to live with it.* Boston: Little Brown.

Carter, V.R. (1980). In retrospect. *Education of the Visually Handicapped, XII* (3), 75–77.

Chong, C. (1992, October). The pitfalls of compliancy. *Braille Monitor,* 542–544.

Cobb, A. (1977). Blindness as an inconvenience: How unwelcome truth becomes "myth." *The Journal of Visual Impairment and Blindness, 71* (9), 406–411.

Columbia Daily Tribune, 1989, March 6. Columbus, MO.

Cott, W. (1973). Evaluation criticizes state school for the blind. In *NAC — correspondence, evasion, and perspective.* Baltimore: National Federation of the Blind.

Crawford, C. H. (1984, November). A question of custodialism follow-up and commentary. *Braille Monitor,* 553–557.

Dewey, J. (1920). *Reconstruction in philosophy.* New York: Henry Holt.

DeWitt, K. (1991, May 12). How best to teach the blind: A growing battle over Braille. *New York Times,* p. 1.

Diamond, C. R. & Petkas, E. (1979). A state agency's view of private-for-profit-rehabilitation. *Journal of Rehabilitation, 45* (3), 30–31.

Dickens, C. (1990/1837). *Oliver Twist.* New York: Bantam.

Dodds, A. G. (1986, July). Mobility: Blind instructors? *Braille Monitor,* 339–343.

Dworkin, R. (1977). *Taking rights seriously.* Cambridge, MA: Harvard University Press.

Eckery, L. L. (1991, December). The everyday usefulness of Braille. *Braille Monitor,* 86–88.

Eisenstadt, S. N. (Ed.). (1968). *Institution building: Ed. papers by Max Weber.* Chicago: University of Chicago Press.

Farrell, G. (1934). Perkins psychological service. *Outlook for the Blind, 28* (2).

Fay, B. (1987). *Critical social science — liberation and its limits.* Ithaca, NY: Cornell University Press.

Foucault, M. (1974). Human nature: Justice versus power. In Elders, F. (Ed.), *Reflective water: Basic concerns of mankind*). London: Souvenir.

——. (1977). *Discipline and punish: The birth of the prison* (A. Sherridan, Trans.). New York: Vintage.

——. (1978). *The history of sexuality* (R. Hurley, Trans.). New York: Pantheon.

Foulke, E. (1972). The personality of the blind: A non-valid concept. *The New Outlook for the Blind, 66* (2), 33–37.

Freidson, E. (1965). Disability as social deviance. In M. B. Sussman (Ed.), *Sociology and rehabilitation* (pp. 71–99). Chicago: The American Sociological Association.

———. (1970). *Profession of medicine: A study of the sociology of applied knowledge.* New York: Dodd and Mead.

French, R. S. (1932). *From Homer to Helen Keller.* New York: American Foundation for the Blind.

Gans, H., Jr. (1973). *More equality.* New York: Pantheon.

Gashel, J. (1984, January). Houston Lighthouse labor contract signed first in the nation's history. *Braille Monitor,* pp. 24–28.

———. (1986, May/June). NFB testifies on workshops. *Braille Monitor,* pp. 256–262.

Gartner, A. (1982, Fall). Images of the disabled/disabling images. *Social Policy, 15.*

Goffman, I. (1961). *Asylums: Essays on the social situation of mental patients and other inmates.* New York: Anchor.

———. (1963). *Stigma: Notes on the management of spoiled identity.* Englewood Cliffs, NJ: Prentice-Hall.

Gomez, P. (1964). Struggle against odds. *The Blind American, 4* (1), 5–6.

Gusfield, J. (1975). Categories of ownership and responsibility in social issues: Alcohol abuse and automobile use. In J. Schneider & J. Kitsuse (Eds.), *Studies in the sociology of social problems.* New Jersey: Ablex.

———. (1982). On the side: Practical action and social constructivism in social problems theory. In J. Schneider & J. Kitsuse (Eds.), *Studies in the sociology of social problems.* New Jersey: Ablex.

———. (1989). Constructing the ownership of social problems: Fun and profit in the welfare state. *Social Problems, 36* (5), 431–441.

Hahn, H. (1990). Theories and values: Ethics and contrasting perspectives on disability. In B. Duncan & D.E. Woods (Eds.), *Ethical issues in disabilities and rehabilitation* (pp. 101–104). New York: World Rehabilitation Fund.

Haug, M. & Sussman, M. B. (1969). Professional autonomy and the revolt of the client. *Social Problems, 17,* 153–167.

Hayes, S. P. (1933). Problems in the psychology of blindness. *Outlook for the Blind, 27* (5), 209.

Hershey, L. (1992, November/December). The 1992 telethon: What happened? *The Disability Rag,* 26–29.

Hodge, C. (1989). Blind workshop workers dealt setback by federal appellate court. *Braille Forum, 1,* 21.

Holsopple, J. Q. (1931). Psychological problems of the newly blinded adult. *Outlook for the Blind, 37* (4).

Ianuzzi, J. (1992, May). Braille or print: Why the debate? *Braille Monitor,* 229–233.

Iowa Commission for the Blind. (n.d.) *What Is the Iowa Commission for the Blind?* Des Moines, IA: State of Iowa.

Irwin, R. (1943). Why rehabilitation of the blind is a function of a special agency for the blind. *Outlook for the Blind, 37* (10).

Jernigan, K. (1965, August). Blindness—concepts and misconceptions. *Braille Monitor,* 76–85.

———. (1968, July). Jacobus tenBroek—the man and the movement. *Braille Monitor,* 29–34.

———. (1970, September). Blindness—the myth and the image. *Braille Monitor,* 117–125.

——. (1973a, February). NAC meets—Blind Demonstrate—Salmon backpeddles. *Braille Monitor,* 126–128.

——. (1973b, January). Partial victory in the NAC battle—and the beat goes on. *Braille Monitor,* 1–26.

——. (1982a, December). Blindness: Handicap or characteristic. *Braille Monitor,* 491–198.

——. (1982b, September). Blindness: Simplicity, complexity, and the public mind. *Braille Monitor,* 374–383.

——. (1984a, March). Electronic canes bring protest from the blind. *Braille Monitor,* 122–126.

——. (1984b, March). Further correspondence about railroads, mass transit and beepers. *Braille Monitor,* 128–133.

——. (1984c, February). Morristown: Comments from a former worker. *Braille Monitor,* 84–86.

——. (1987, September). The National Braille Association cuts its ties with NAC. *Braille Monitor,* 326–328.

——. (1988a, May/June). Editorial comment preceding C. Brown, The Richmond workshop: Bad management, "quality service," and NAC. *Braille Monitor,* 228–229.

——. (1988b, September/October). A thought-provoking resolution and an issue which is not yet settled. *Braille Monitor,* 462–465.

——. (1989, June). Blind workers claim wages exploitive. *Braille Monitor,* 322.

——. (1990, February). Consumerism: Improving the service delivery system. (In a speech given at the Penn-Del Chapter of the Association for Education and Rehabilitation of the Blind and Visually Impaired in Lancaster, PA, Nov. 17, 1989). *Braille Monitor,* 102–106.

——. (1991a, January). Honor roll of pride: A list of agencies which have withdrawn from NAC accreditation. *Braille Monitor,* 40–41.

——. (1991b, September). NAC in the death throes: The passing of an era. *Braille Monitor,* 458–466.

——. (1991c, January). NAC: What price accreditation. *Braille Monitor,* 17–4.

——. (1991d, January). Roll call of shame: A list of NAC accredited organizations. *Braille Monitor,* pp. 30–40.

Johnson, T.J. (1967). *Professions and power.* London: Macmillan.

Katz, M. B. (1986). *In the shadow of the poorhouse: A sociological history of welfare in America* (2nd ed.). New York: Basic Books.

Kiesler, C. A. (1992, September). U.S. mental health policy: Doomed to fail. *American Psychologist,* 1077–1081.

Kirchner, C. (1983a). Statistical Brief Number 24, private agencies serving blind and visually impaired persons—a survey of funding and staffing: Part I. *Journal of Visual Impairment and Blindness, 77* (8), 400–403.

——. (1983b). Statistical Brief Number 25, private agencies serving blind and visually impaired persons—a survey of funding and staffing: Part II. *Journal of Visual Impairment and Blindness, 77* (9), 451–455.

Kirtley, D. D. (1975). *The psychology of blindness.* Chicago: Nelson-Hall.

Koestler, F. A. (1976). *The unseen minority — A social history of blindness in America.* New York: David McKay.

Lane, H. (1992). *The mask of benevolence: Disabling the deaf community.* New York: Alfred A. Knopf.

Larson, M. S. (1977). *The rise of professionalism: A sociological analysis.* Berkeley: University of California Press.

Lewin, S. S., Ramsuer, J. H. & Fink, J. M. (1979). The role of private rehabilitation: Founder, catalyst, competition. *Journal of Rehabilitation, 45* (3), 15–19.

Lipsky, M. (1980). *Street level bureaucracy.* New York: Russell Sage.

Longmore, P. K. (1985). Screening stereotypes: Images of disabled people. *Social Policy, 16* (1), 31–37.

Lowenfeld, B. (1944). Psychological principles in home teaching. *Outlook for the Blind, 38* (2), 32–35.

——. (1947). Psychological aspects of blindness. *Outlook for the Blind, 41* (2).

——. (1962). Psychological foundation of special methods in teaching blind children. In P. A. Zahl (Ed.), *Blindness — modern approaches to the unseen environment.* New York: Hafner.

——. (1963). Psychological problems of children with impaired vision. In E. W. Cruchshank (Ed.), *Psychology of exceptional children and youth* (2nd ed.). Englewood Cliffs, NJ: Prentice Hall.

——. (1975). *The changing status of the blind: From separation to integration.* Springfield, IL: Charles C Thomas, Publisher.

Mannheim, K. (1936). *Ideology and utopia: An introduction to the sociology of knowledge.* (L. Wirth and E. Shils, Trans.). New York: Harcourt Brace.

Matras, J. (1990). *Dependency, obligations and entitlements.* New Jersey: Prentice Hall.

Matson, F. W. (1963). California sheltered shop ousts blind workers. *The Blind American, 3* (5), 3–4.

——. (1990). *Walking alone and marching together: A history of the organized blind movement in the United States, 1940-1990.* Baltimore: National Federation of the Blind.

Maurer, M. (1989, October). Presidential report: Language and the future of the blind. *Braille Monitor,* 576–588.

——. (1991, July/August). Who should learn Braille and why? *Braille Monitor,* pp. 360–361.

McConnell, D. (1978, January). NAC and consumers. *Braille Monitor,* 1–15.

Megivern, K. (1991). To dissolve or not to dissolve . . . NAC members say "NO!" *AER Report, 8* (3), 2–5.

Mettler, R. (1987). Blindness and managing the environment. *Journal of Visual Impairment and Blindness, 81* (10), 476–481.

Minnesota Department of Jobs and Training Services for the Blind and Visually Impaired. (1992). Individualized Written Rehabilitation Program for Jennifer Lehman.

Mizruchi, E. H. (1983). *Regulating society: Marginality and social control in historical perspective.* New York: Free Press.

Moore, B. (1966). *Social origins of dictatorship and democracy.* Boston: Beacon.

Mulholland, M. E. (1992). Prologue. *Journal of Visual Impairment and Blindness, 86* (7), 309–314.

National Accreditation Council Annual Report. (1968).

National Federation of the Blind of Minnesota. (n.d.). *Minnesota Programs for the blind: Training facilities effectiveness survey,* (Summary edition). Minneapolis, MN.

Olson, C. (1977). Blindness can be reduced to an inconvenience. *Journal of Visual Impairment and Blindness, 71* (9), 406–411.

———. (1981). Paper barriers. *Journal of Visual Impairment and Blindness, 75* (8), 338–339.

Omvig, J. (1983, March). What we can expect from a commission for the blind viewpoint from the consumers. *Braille Monitor,* 86–92.

———. (1983, July). Are we blind, or something else? What's in a word? *Braille Monitor,* 227–232.

Organist, J. (1979). Private sector rehabilitation: Benefits, dangers, and implications for education. *Journal of Rehabilitation, 45* (3), 56–58.

Organization for Social and Technical Innovation, Inc. (1971). *Blindness and services to the blind.* Cambridge, MA: OSTI Press.

Outlook for the Blind. (1941). News and views of the A.A.W.B. *Outlook for the Blind, 35,* 4.

Outlook for the Blind. (1942). News and views of the A.A.W.B. *Outlook for the Blind, 36,* 3.

Pierce, B. (1991a, September). A new way out: Iowa School for the Blind de-NACs. *Braille Monitor,* 500–501.

———. (1991b, February). Editorial preface to: The proof of the pudding. *Braille Monitor,* 102–103.

———. (1991c, March). What's in an attitude? *Braille Monitor,* 159–162.

Pinder, P. (1991, September). NAC at 25: A look at the numbers. *Braille Monitor,* 25–30.

Randall, C. H. (1989, August). Blind: Then and now. *Braille Monitor,* 466–467.

Richardson, S. A., et al. (1961). Cultural uniformity in reaction to physical disabilities. *American Sociological Review, 26,* 241–247.

Rothman, D. J. (1971). *The Discovery of the asylum: Social order and disorder in the new republic.* Boston: Little, Brown.

———. (1978). The state as parent. In W. Gaylin, et al (Eds.), *Doing good* (pp. 69–92). New York: Pantheon.

Rothman, D. & Rothman, S.M. (1984). *The Willowbrook Wars.* New York: Harper & Row.

Rousseau, J. (1979/1762). *Emile: or, on education* (Allan Bloom, Trans.). New York: Basic Books.

Santin & Simmons. (1977). Problems in the construction of reality in congenitally blind children. *Journal of Visual Impairment and Blindness, 71* (10), 425–429.

Scanlan, T. (1990). *Summary of Training Effectiveness Survey.* Minnesota State Services for the Blind.

Schama, S. (1989). *Citizens.* New York: Vintage.

Schneider, Joseph W. (1985). Social problems theory: The constructionist view. In R.H. Turner (Ed.), *Annual Review of Sociology, 11,* 209–229.

Schroeder, F. (1992, June). Braille bills: What are they and what do they mean? *Braille Monitor*, 308–311.

Schulz, P. (1977). Who says blindness is just an inconvenience? *Journal of Visual Impairment and Blindness, 71* (5), 230–231.

Schuster, C. S. 1986. Sex education of the visually impaired child: The role of parents. *Journal of Visual Impairment and Blindness, 80* (4), 675–680.

Scott, R. A. (1967). The factory as a social service organization: Goal displacement in workshops for the blind. *Social Problems, 15* (2), 160–175.

——. (1969). *The making of blind men: A study of adult socialization.* New York: Russell Sage.

Selvin, H. (1976). How to succeed at being blind. *New Outlook for the Blind, 70* (10), 420–428.

Sidis, H. (1944). Concerning attitudes of the blind. *Outlook for the Blind, 38* (2),

Siberman, Ken. (1991, February). The proof of the pudding. *Braille Monitor*, 102–103.

Sjoberg, G., Brymer, R. A., & Farris, B. (1966). Bureaucracy and the lower class. *Sociology and social research, 50*, 325–337.

Smith, A. (1976/1759). *The theory of moral sentiments.* D. Raphael and A. Macfie (Eds.). Oxford: Clarendon.

——. (1976/1776). *The wealth of nations.* New York: Oxford University Press.

Spector, M. & Kitsuse, J. I. (1977). *Constructing social programs.* Melno Park, CA: Cummings.

——. (1987). *Constructing social problems.* New York: Aldine De Gryter.

Stein, J. (1967, November 19). Blindness study urged by doctor. *New York Times.* p. 19.

Stetten, D. Jr. (1981). Coping with Blindness. *New England Journal of Medicine, 30* (8), 458–460.

Sussman, M. B. (1969). Dependent disabled and dependent poor: Similarity of conceptual issues and research needs. *The Social Service Review, 43*, 383–395.

Swaan, A. D. (1990). *The management of normality.* London and New York: Routledge.

tenBroek, J. (1948, October). A bill of rights for the blind. *Outlook for the Blind.*

——. (1951). *The antislavery origins of the 14th Amendment.* Berkeley: University of California Press.

——. (1955). *The Constitution and the right of free movement.* New York: National Travelers Aid Association.

——. (1962, May). The character and function of sheltered workshops. *The Blind American*, 19–29.

——. (1965a, July). Agency conference on standards set. *Braille Monitor*, 28–29.

——. (1965b, August). The Federation at twenty-five: Postview and preview. *Braille Monitor*, 86–93.

——. (1966a, June). COMSTAC's children—the instruments of accreditation. *Braille Monitor*, 15–19.

——. (1966b). Letter to Arthur L. Brandon. In *NAC—Correspondence, Evasion, and Perspective.* Des Moines: National Federation of the Blind.

——. (1966c, July). NFB—COMSTAC differences aired. *Braille Monitor*, 21–28.

——. (1967, July). Blindness insuperable says Stanford. *Braille Monitor*, 402–409.

tenBroek, J., Barnhart, E. N., & Matson, F. (1968). *Prejudice, war and the Constitution.* Berkeley: University of California Press.

tenBroek, J., & Handler, J.F. (Eds.). (1971). *Family law and the poor: Essays.* Westport, CT: Greenwood.

tenBroek, J. and Matson, F. (1959). *Hope deferred: Public welfare and the blind.* Berkeley: University of California Press.

——. (1966a, March). COMSTAC—the clients' big brother. *Braille Monitor,* 45–51.

——. (1966b, January). COMSTAC's standards for vocational services. *Braille Monitor,* 8–10.

——. (1966c, February). Note on authors. *Braille Monitor,* 1.

Twaddle, A. (1973). Illness and deviance. *Social Science and Medicine, 7,* 751–762.

Tuttle, D. W. (1984). *Self esteem and adjusting to blindness: The process of responding to life's demands.* Springfield, IL: Charles C Thomas, Publisher.

——. (1986). Family members responding to visual impairment. *Education of the Visually Handicapped, XVIII* (3), 107–116.

United States Department of Education. (1992a). People with Disabilities in Basic Life Activities in the United States. *Disability Statistics Abstract* (#3, April). Washington, DC: U.S. Government Printing Office.

United States Department of Education. (1992b). People with Work Disabilities in the United States. *Disability Statistics Abstract* (#4, May). Washington, DC: U.S. Government Printing Office.

Vaughan, C. E. (1990, June). What went wrong with doing good. *Braille Monitor,* 362–365.

——. (1991). The social basis of conflict between blind people and agents of rehabilitation. *Disability, Handicap & Society, 6,* (3), 203–217.

——. (1992a). The development of public policy and new laws concerning the rights of disabled persons in the People's Republic of China. (in press). *The Journal of Disabilities Studies.*

——. *(1992b, JanuaryFebruary). Why I am still a Federationist. Disability Rag,* 40–41.

——. (1993, in press). New images for the blindness system. *Journal of Rehabilitation, 59* (1).

Vaughan, C. E., & Vaughan, J. (accepted for publication in 1993). The decline in autonomy for blind workers in China. *Review.*

Vaughan, T. R., Sjoberg, G., & Rynolds, L.T. (Eds.). (1993). *A critique of contemporary American sociology.* Dix Hills, NY: General Hall.

Walhof, R. (1984, October). Rehabilitation for the blind: Patterns, problems and options. *Braille Monitor,* pp. 459–467.

Walker, D. L. (1974). Accreditation or evaluation. *Education of the Visually Handicapped, VI* (4), 125–126.

——. (1975). Don't be silly, I'm your other end! *Education of the Visually Handicapped, VII* (2), 63–64.

Walter, G. A. (1984). Organizational development and individual rights. *The Journal of Applied Behavioral Science, 20* (4), 423–439.

Walton, J. (1990). *Sociology and critical inquiry: The work, tradition, and purpose* (2nd ed.). Belmont, CA: Wadsworth.

Weaver, C. L. (1991, July/August). Vocational rehabilitation reform: Holding out a hand? *American Enterprise,* 20–23.

Weber, M. (1978/1920). *Economy and society* (G. Roth, Trans.). New York: Bedminster.

Webson, A. (1992, July). *Access.* Keynote address at international Council for Education of the Visually Handicapped Ninth Quinquennial Conference. Bangkok, Thailand.

Wiener, W. et al. (1992). Report of consumer work group. *Journal of Visual Impairment and Blindness, 86* (7), 349–353.

Wilensky, H.L. (1964). The professionalization of everyone? *American Journal of Sociology LXX* (2), 137–158.

Wilson, J. (1992). The freedom bell. In K. Jernigan (Ed.), *The freedom bell* (pp. 33–43). Baltimore, MD: National Federation of the Blind.

Wolfe, A. (1989). *Whose keeper? Social science and moral obligation.* Berkeley: University of California Press.

Wright, B. A. (1988). Attitudes and the fundamental negative bias—conditions and corrections. In H. Yukev (Ed.), *Attitudes towards persons with disabilities* (pp. 1–21). New York: Springer.

York, Robert. (1991, November 12). *Vocational rehabilitation program client characteristics, services received, and employment outcomes.* Testimony before the Commission on Education and Labor, House of Representatives.

Yukev, H. (1988). *Attitudes towards persons with disabilities.* New York: Springer.

Zola, I. K. (1983). Toward independent living: Goals and dilemmas. In N.M. Crewe and I. K. Zola (Eds.), *Independent living for physically disabled people.* San Francisco: Jossey-Bass.

NAME INDEX

SUBJECT INDEX